THE EVERYTHING GUIDE TO NUTRITION

Dear Reader,

Throughout my professional and personal experience in health and wellness, I have discovered that simple changes in diet and lifestyle can have a tremendous impact. But determining how to make those changes can be overwhelming, and nutritional guidance can be extremely valuable. It's not an all-or-nothing situation when it comes to finding your body's balance. A few shifts in food choices and behavior can help you increase your energy levels, control your hunger, and manage your health.

Life presents challenges. Busy schedules, providing meals, and enjoying a social life can make it difficult to think of eating for energy. After seeing many of my clients get overwhelmed with meal plans, food shopping, label reading, and recipes during their quest for wellness, it became clear that they needed simple tools to guide them through their journey. Many people have an idea of how to make better food choices, but with more than 15,000 new food products being introduced into our food supply every year—and the marketing gimmicks that go along with them—frustration and confusion can result. Additionally, every day we hear about new fad diets that sidetrack us and prevent us from learning more about basic nutrition.

I hope this book will give you an abundance of ideas about what to eat that is delicious, easy to make, and provides the energy you need. You'll learn small changes you can apply every day to improve your life. It's time to let go of all those negative connections to food and rebuild an incredible and manageable experience for your health.

Yours in good health,

Nicole Cormier, RD, LDN

Welcome to the EVERYTHING® Series!

These handy, accessible books give you all you need to tackle a difficult project, gain a new hobby, comprehend a fascinating topic, prepare for an exam, or even brush up on something you learned back in school but have since forgotten.

You can choose to read an *Everything®* book from cover to cover or just pick out the information you want from our four useful boxes: e-questions, e-facts, e-alerts, and e-ssentials.

We give you everything you need to know on the subject, but throw in a lot of fun stuff along the way, too.

We now have more than 400 *Everything®* books in print, spanning such wide-ranging categories as weddings, pregnancy, cooking, music instruction, foreign language, crafts, pets, New Age, and so much more. When you're done reading them all, you can finally say you know *Everything®*!

QUESTION

Answers to
common questions

FACT

Important snippets
of information

ALERT

Urgent
warnings

ESSENTIAL

Quick
handy tips

PUBLISHER Karen Cooper

DIRECTOR OF ACQUISITIONS AND INNOVATION Paula Munier

MANAGING EDITOR, EVERYTHING® SERIES Lisa Laing

COPY CHIEF Casey Ebert

ACQUISITIONS AND DEVELOPMENT EDITOR Katrina Schroeder

EDITORIAL ASSISTANT Ross Weisman

EVERYTHING® SERIES COVER DESIGNER Erin Alexander

LAYOUT DESIGNERS Colleen Cunningham, Elisabeth Lariviere, Ashley Vierra, Denise Wallace

THE EVERYTHING®

GUIDE TO NUTRITION

All you need to keep you—and
your family—healthy

Nicole Cormier, RD, LDN

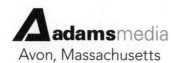

Avon, Massachusetts

Dedicated to my family and friends who have supported my projects, workshops, and career over the years

An Everything® Series Book.
Everything® and everything.com® are registered trademarks of F+W Media, Inc.

Published by Adams Media, a division of F+W Media, Inc.
57 Littlefield Street, Avon, MA 02322 U.S.A.
www.adamsmedia.com

This book contains material adapted and abridged from: *The Everything® Cooking for Kids Cookbook; The Everything® Diabetes Cookbook; The Everything® Family Nutrition Book; The Everything® Food Allergy Cookbook; The Everything® Guide to Being Vegetarian; The Everything® Guide to Macrobiotics; The Everything® Healthy College Cookbook; The Everything® Healthy Slow Cooker Cookbook; The Everything® Low-fat, High Flavor Cookbook; The Everything® Nutrition Book; The Everything® Organic Cooking for Baby and Toddler Book; The Everything® Raw Food Recipe Book; The Everything® Superfoods Book; The Everything® Vegan Cookbook; The Everything® Vegetarian Cookbook.*

ISBN 10: 1-4405-1030-X
ISBN 13: 978-1-4405-1030-4
eISBN 10: 1-4405-1159-4
eISBN 13: 978-1-4405-1159-2

Printed in the United States of America.

10 9 8 7 6 5 4 3 2

Library of Congress Cataloging-in-Publication Data
Cormier, Nicole.
The everything guide to nutrition / Nicole Cormier.
p. cm.
Includes bibliographical references and index.
ISBN 978-1-4405-1030-4 (alk. paper)
1. Nutrition. 2. Health. 3. Food habits. I. Title.
RA784.C595   2011
613.2—dc22   2010039142

Contents

Acknowledgments

I would like to give a special thanks to all the clients and patients I've had the opportunity to work with during the past five years. You've truly inspired me to continue my career as a registered dietitian and nutrition counselor. I am so grateful to have been a part of each of your journeys toward a healthier lifestyle.

Top 10 Reasons Why Understanding Basic Nutrition Can Improve Your Life

1. Basic nutrition focuses on regulating blood sugars, which is important in managing your energy levels, hunger, and weight.

2. Consuming nutrient-dense unprocessed foods without added solid fats, sugars, starches, or sodium can improve and prevent chronic diseases.

3. Lifestyle changes alone can decrease, or even eliminate, the need for several medications related to cholesterol levels, blood pressure, diabetes, and depression, resulting in fewer side effects.

4. Many lifestyle changes modify contributors to cardiovascular disease, such as high blood pressure, high blood sugar, and obesity. Therefore, changing your life can certainly save your life.

5. Eating foods such as beans and quinoa, two "superfoods" that provide both protein and fiber, can help you regulate your blood sugars, hunger, and energy levels.

6. Fats can prevent vitamin deficiencies and create satiety in your life. Polyunsaturated and monounsaturated fats from nuts, oils, avocados, and olives are essential for absorbing fat-soluble vitamins A, D, E, and K.

7. Many processed foods cause your pancreas to work more than twice as hard as it should. Today, about 18 million Americans have diabetes and 41 million are pre-diabetic.

8. The average American consumes 6,000–18,000 mg of sodium per day, which can result in high blood pressure, heart disease, fluid retention, and stroke.

9. Despite government labeling requirements, food companies use multiple and sometimes confusing schemes to attract consumers to their products.

10. Fiber sustains a healthy digestive system; however, isolated fiber (the fiber food manufactures add to foods that would otherwise not contain fiber) is not equivalent to whole fiber.

Introduction

WE ARE WHAT WE eat. The old saying still holds true today for busy people trying to find balance in their overworked, overstressed lives. Many of us have little time to manage meals, energy levels, and a lifestyle path toward whole health. The idea of basic nutrition and eating for energy seems to have become an inconvenient thought in our everyday lives. Perhaps we feel overwhelmed by the abundance of foods available to us, the quick-fix diets calling our names, or the confusion between true energy sources that increase our performance and random spikes in our blood sugars that cause us to crave more sugar.

It is easy to understand why the rate of heart disease, diabetes, cancer, and stroke has increased so rapidly in recent decades when you consider that some of the most common foods consumed in the United States are processed with added solid fats, sugars, starches, and sodium. In most cases, micronutrients that were lost during processing are added or replaced later. You may be thinking: Why in the world would we go through so much trouble to break down our foods from their natural states, then enrich them with nutrients that may be less absorbable by the time they are in our digestive systems, especially when these foods are contributing to the rise in obesity and chronic illnesses? It makes sense that we will have poor health if we eat foods with poor nutritional value.

According to the National Cancer Institute, 90–95 percent of Americans exceed the recommended consumption of refined grains, which are defined as a grain product that lacks the bran, germ, or endosperm. Therefore, they provide little nutrition. These foods are culprits that entice us in the most convenient ways: in fast-food drive-thrus, vending machines, and packages that can stay on supermarket shelves for long periods of time.

If you read every piece of information on a product's Nutrition Fact Label and are still confused as to whether or not it is a good food choice, you may realize how inferior products are slipping past even discerning consumers. The Nutrition Labeling laws have changed several times over the years, allowing marketing departments to give consumers a run for their money. Many new products that reach supermarket shelves each year are non–nutrient-dense foods, which have few natural micronutrients and lots of "empty calories."

The *Everything*® *Guide to Nutrition* is about eating real, whole, delicious food, but it goes beyond just handing over a meal plan. People have a desperate need to understand basic nutrition to help them feel their best, mentally and physically. Focusing on lifestyle changes instead of following a specific diet is the ticket to achieving optimal health, decreasing your risk of illness, increasing your energy level, improving your quality of life and well-being, and reducing your medications.

Multiple factors block us from transitioning into a healthier population. One solution may be to restructure our food choices from the ground up, consuming fewer processed foods. As you read this book, keep an open mind about new foods that are waiting to support your health in many ways. The support they offer will give you a new appreciation of and positive relationship with foods that provide your body with the energy it needs to perform. This book is about understanding how to eat for energy and live mindfully, instead of just following a trend.

CHAPTER 1

Healthy Measures

A healthy lifestyle isn't a one-size-fits-all affair. Each person needs to discover what practices are right for him or her and incorporate them into everyday life in order to achieve long-term success. No matter what outcomes you desire— weight loss, more energy, lower cholesterol, or a healthier digestive system—finding your own starting point is a crucial part of beginning your personal journey to wellness. It's time to let go of fad diets and take the wheel. You have the ability to assess where you're at and where you want to go, and now you'll learn how to get there.

Dietary Guidelines

The U.S. Department of Agriculture (USDA) and the U.S. Department of Health and Human Services (HHS) first created the Dietary Guidelines for Americans in 1980. Revisions are made every five years and can be accessed at *www .health.gov/dietaryguidelines/history.htm*. These guidelines were designed to teach people what to eat to stay healthy. They reflect the most up-to-date and sound nutritional information known about healthy eating and a healthy lifestyle. The guidelines provide nutrition advice about choosing and preparing foods, as well as about living an active lifestyle that will help promote health and prevent disease. The Dietary Guidelines for Americans apply to all healthy Americans over the age of two. They focus on health promotion and risk reduction, and also form the basis of federal food, nutrition education, and information programs. The guidelines include specific recommendations that carry three basic messages: aim for fitness, build a healthy base, and choose sensibly. They provide these key recommendations for the general public:

- Choose a variety of foods from the basic food groups that are nutrient dense.
- Limit saturated fats and trans fats, cholesterol, added sugars, sodium, and alcohol consumption.
- Balance caloric intake with calories expended through physical activity to manage a healthy weight.
- Aim for at least thirty minutes of moderate-intensity physical activity per day on most days of the week to promote physical health, optimal body weight, and mental health.
- Consume a variety of at least 2 cups of fruit and 2½ cups of vegetables per day.
- Consume 3 ounces or more (depending on your goals) of whole grains per day.
- Use low-fat or nonfat dairy products as a protein source. Consume about 3 cups per day.
- Saturated fats should make up less than 10 percent of daily calories.
- Trans fats should be consumed in as limited quantities as possible.
- Cholesterol intake should be less than 300 milligrams per day.

- Most fats should come from polyunsaturated and monounsaturated sources such as fish, nuts, and vegetable oils. Keep calories from fat between 20 and 35 percent of daily calories.
- Choose lean proteins from beans, nuts, seeds, dairy products, fish, eggs, poultry, pork, and red meat.
- Eat high-fiber foods such as fruits, vegetables, and whole grains several times per day.
- Consume small amounts of added sugars or other sweeteners.
- Consume less than 2,300 milligrams of sodium per day.
- Limit alcoholic beverages to one drink or less per day for women and two drinks or less per day for men. This recommendation does not apply to people who cannot restrict alcohol intake, pregnant or lactating women, children and adolescents, persons on medications that could interact with alcohol, or those with any specific medical condition that might be exacerbated by alcohol consumption.

The 2010 Dietary Guidelines focus on eating a healthy, plant-based diet, developing a positive relationship with food, and being a cautious and mindful eater. Eat foods, not just nutrients, and savor your food as well as the process of cooking it. The guidelines also emphasize prevention and kid-specific awareness, the value of eating seafood outweighing the risks, and nourishing your body no matter what you weigh.

Assessing Your Weight

When evaluating your weight, you need to consider various factors. Body weight should not be the only method used in assessing your weight and health. Body weight alone does not convey how much body fat you have or where it is stored—the strongest predictors of health risk. It is important to know how much of your weight is body fat, where that body fat is located, and whether you already have health problems related to your weight. A number of assessment methods can be used to determine whether a person is at a healthy weight. Some of these are based on height and weight, others are based on measurements of body fat. The general idea is to determine whether your weight puts you at risk for health problems so you can take action if necessary.

FACT

To properly weigh yourself, weigh on the same scale each time you weigh in. Use a beam balance scale, not a spring scale, whenever possible. Be sure the scale is periodically calibrated for accuracy. Wear lightweight clothing, and do not wear shoes. For consistency, try to weigh yourself at the same time of day each time (morning is best).

Your body shape can be used in assessing your weight. Where you store body fat can be an indication of a healthy weight and health status. Are you an "apple" shape, storing excess body fat in the stomach area and around the waist? An apple shape can put you at higher risk for health problems such as early heart disease, high blood pressure, Type 2 diabetes, and certain types of cancer. Are you a "pear" shape, storing excess body fat below the waist, in the hips, buttocks, and thighs? A pear shape does not appear to be as harmful to a person's health as an apple shape.

If you cannot tell by looking at your body in the mirror whether you are an apple or a pear shape, you can figure your waist-to-hip ratio. Follow these steps to figure out your waist-to-hip ratio.

1. Use a ninety-six-inch tape measure.
2. Stand relaxed. Measure your waist at its smallest point without sucking in your stomach.
3. Measure your hips at the largest part of your buttocks and hips.
4. Divide your waist measurement by your hip measurement.
5. If this number is nearly or more than 1.0, you would be considered an apple shape.
6. If this number is considerably less than 1.0, you would be considered a pear shape.

▼ **Where Does Your Waist-To-Hip Measurement Fall?**

Health Risk	Men	Women
High Risk	>1.0	>0.85
Moderately High Risk	0.90–1.0	0.80–0.85
Low Risk	<0.90	<0.80

Weighing Your Risk

Carrying around extra weight every day can be a heavy burden and a health risk. Every system in the body needs to work harder to cope with that weight. Being overweight is defined as having an excess amount of body weight that includes muscle, bone, fat, and water. Being obese specifically refers to having an excess amount of body fat. Bodybuilders or athletes with a lot of muscle can be overweight without being obese. Obesity occurs when a person consumes more calories than she burns.

As dangerous as it is to carry around extra weight, being underweight is associated with a higher mortality rate. Being underweight can lead to the malfunctioning of many important body functions. It can also result in a loss of energy and an increased susceptibility to injury, infection, and illness. The causes of being over- or underweight can be complex, and they differ among individuals. Genetics, environment, social, behavioral, and psychological reasons can all be factors in an abnormal body weight. You may not be able to change some of these factors, but one you can change is your lifestyle habits.

The Health Hazards of Obesity

Losing just 5 to 10 percent of excess body weight can help to reduce your risk for health problems related to your weight. A small loss in body weight can help lower blood pressure, total cholesterol, LDL cholesterol (bad cholesterol), triglyceride levels, and blood sugar. Lifestyle change is the healthiest and most permanent method of losing weight and decreasing the risk of serious health problems. Combining a healthy diet with increased physical activity and behavior modification is the most successful strategy for weight loss and healthy weight maintenance.

Obesity can generate stress, both physically and emotionally. It can lead to feelings of low self-esteem as well as social seclusion. Since 1985, obesity has been recognized as a chronic disease. It is the second leading cause of preventable death, surpassed only by cigarette smoking. Physical health problems related to obesity include heart disease, Type 2 diabetes, high blood cholesterol levels, high blood pressure, stroke, gallbladder disease, liver disease, osteoarthritis, gout, pulmonary problems, and certain types of cancer.

Your Ideal Weight

Our country as a whole is overweight. The American lifestyle has evolved into a sedentary pattern, with many people engaging in virtually no physical activity. Most Americans drive to work and sit at computers, then drive home and sit in front of their televisions. Kids get driven to school, where they sit all day, until they come home and sit at their computers, TVs, or video games.

Meanwhile the supermarkets are packed with cheap, good-tasting, high-calorie foods. Coffee shops wait at every corner to give us a boost of artificial energy in the form of caffeine and sugar. The fast-food companies are conveniently located in our markets, shopping malls, and airports. They even supply our schools with lunches. It's no wonder a majority of Americans are overweight.

The technology of underdeveloped countries is not at our level, but neither is their rate of obesity. When people from those parts of the world immigrate to the West, their rate of weight gain quickly catches up to ours.

QUESTION

How did people get so fat in the first place?
The human body was designed to enjoy and consume as much high-calorie food as possible. Humans are built to store extra calories in pockets of fat until needed during winter or a time of famine. Unfortunately, human physiology has not compensated for technological advances.

Consequences of Being Overweight

Overweight people run higher risks for heart disease, high blood pressure, osteoporosis, osteoarthritis, infertility, stroke, diabetes, and numerous forms of cancer. Obesity is about to pass tobacco as the leading cause of preventable death.

Regardless of how your weight compares to a table or chart, you know if you and your family need to pay more attention to nutrition. An ideal weight is one that you can maintain, that allows you to be active, enables you to have energy throughout the day, and lets you sleep at night. What works for some does not necessarily work for all. You are an individual, and it's your unique lifestyle that determines your overall weight and health.

Where do you and your family fit in to this scenario? Are you physically active? Are you at a healthy weight? There are specific measurements you can make to determine exactly where you stand (see Appendix B), but you probably have a pretty good idea already.

Battle of the Bulge

If you determine that you need to lose weight, there is only one way to do it. You must burn more calories than you consume. There are dozens of diet plans, programs, pills, and shakes vying for your dollar. But the only healthy way to lose those excess pounds is by controlling portion sizes, understanding which foods your body needs, and incorporating exercise into your daily routine.

Cutting calories takes attention, and burning them takes effort. There's no getting around it.

You can lose about a pound a week if you eliminate or burn 500 calories a day. To help you gauge this, an 8-ounce container of low-fat, plain yogurt has about 150 calories. People who run regularly burn about 100 calories per mile. Eat less, exercise more. Sounds simple enough, right?

What Are Calories?

To understand how to achieve and maintain a healthy weight, you need to start with your calorie needs. It is possible to manage your weight by balancing the calories you eat and the physical activities you choose. Calories measure the amount of energy in foods. Your body relies on calories to keep you alive and functioning.

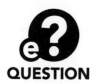

QUESTION

How many calories do nutrients provide?
Carbohydrates, protein, and fat are the only three nutrients that provide calories in food. Fat provides nine calories per gram, carbohydrates provide four calories per gram, and protein provides four calories per gram.

Three nutrients in foods provide calories, or energy: carbohydrates, protein, and fat. These nutrients are released from food during the digestive process, and then absorbed into the bloodstream and converted to glucose or blood sugar. Glucose is your body's main source of energy.

Your Body's Calorie Needs

Your body constantly needs calories, or energy, to maintain its basic functions. Having a general idea of your body's total calorie needs can help you to maintain, lose, or gain weight. Everyone's caloric needs differ, depending on factors such as age, gender, size, body composition, basal metabolic rate, and physical activity.

Basal metabolic rate (BMR) is the rate at which your body burns calories when at rest. It is the level of energy your body needs to keep your normal body processes going, such as heartbeat, breathing, body temperature, and transmitting messages to your brain. Your BMR uses up 60 percent of your body's total energy needs.

Estimating Your Calorie Needs

There are different methods for estimating caloric needs for individuals. Though just an estimate, the BMR can give you a general idea of how many calories your body needs. Whether you are overweight, at your healthy weight, or underweight, it is important to know how many calories you should be consuming for good health and to reach or maintain a healthy weight. The following simple equation can help you easily estimate your caloric needs:

1. Figure your BMR by multiplying your healthy weight (in pounds) by 10 for women and 11 for men. If you are overweight, use the average weight within the range given on the BMI in Appendix B. Using your actual weight, if you are overweight, will overestimate your calorie needs.
2. Figure your calorie needs for physical activity. Multiply your BMR, from step 1, by the percentage that matches your activity level: sedentary, 20 percent; light activity, 30 percent; moderate activity, 40 percent; very active, 50 percent.

3. Add calories needed for digestion and absorption of nutrients in your body. Add your calories for BMR, from step 1, and your calories for physical activity, from step 2, then multiply the total by 10 percent.
4. Total your calorie needs by adding the calories from each step.

Serving Sizes

The Food Group Pyramid provides a suggested range of the number of servings you should eat each day from each food group. The number of servings and the size of the servings you eat comprise your daily caloric intake.

ESSENTIAL

If you are a vegetarian, you can still make the Food Guide Pyramid work for you. A vegetarian who completely avoids meat, poultry, and fish can choose alternate foods from the meat group. Some of these alternate choices include peanut butter, dry beans or peas, eggs, nuts, and soy foods such as tofu, tempeh, veggie burgers, and soy milk. Use peanut butter and nuts sparingly because they tend to be high in fat.

Keep in mind that serving sizes are only approximations. If you do not have any idea of what a serving size should look like, it would be a good idea to start measuring your foods. Once you have an idea of what a serving should look like, it will be easier to eye your portion sizes in the future.

For mixed foods, such as pizza, do your best to estimate the food group servings contained in the food. For example, a slice of pizza can be counted as the grain group for the crust, the milk group for the cheese, and the vegetable group for the tomato sauce. Toppings such as Canadian bacon or pepperoni would count as a meat. Mushrooms would count in the vegetable group.

CHAPTER 2

The Ideal Diet

The word "diet" has been used tirelessly over the years, in most cases meaning a regimen of eating to reduce weight. This approach has mostly created short-term success in reaching weight-loss goals. But without a solid foundation, temporary behavior changes dissolve relatively quickly and dieters fall back into old patterns. Perhaps, looking at "diet" as habitual nourishment could create a more positive environment for long-term changes. Knowing what you should be eating, instead of what you shouldn't, and understanding how eating an ideal diet would improve your life will boost your momentum.

Balance

Life balance involves a combination of body balance, work balance, family balance, and social balance. Body balance itself has several parts that are necessary to make it achievable. To fuel your metabolism and motivate yourself to participate in daily activities you need to manage your daily food intake, balancing your calories in and your calories out. You also need balance among the food groups you consume at each meal, the time between meals, and the rate at which digestion occurs.

Ninety-five percent of calories should come from vegetables and fruits, protein, whole grains, and healthy fats. The remaining 5 percent can come from food that has less nutritional value. This creates a balance of your caloric distribution throughout the day.

If you understand basic nutrition, you can achieve optimal health by managing your blood sugars, energy levels, and hunger throughout the day. One way to do this is by eating a small meal or snack every three to four hours.

Most meals should be divided so that more than half of your plate contains vegetables and/or fruit and the remainder a lean protein and whole grain. A protein and a fiber should be present at each meal. These combinations make it possible for you to physically feel full and experience satiety. They work together to slow your digestion and prevent your blood sugar from increasing or falling dramatically. Learning to put these combinations together at each meal and most snacks will help keep blood sugars at a balanced level, which will reduce hunger. It will also prevent you from feeling cranky, sleepy, and starving.

Superfoods

Superfoods are particular types of food that contain high amounts of phytonutrients, necessary for the proper functioning of the body. Individually, they provide important health benefits, but taken as a whole they become a major defense against the ravages of free radicals, environmental toxins, and heavy-metal contamination. You can find numerous articles on the benefits of foods considered to be "super," and it seems everyone has their favorites. Twenty foods are almost unanimously found on all the superfood lists. They are:

1. Apples (fight free radicals)
2. Blueberries (most antioxidants ever)
3. Broccoli (helps prevent cancer)
4. Quinoa (the mother grain)
5. Dark chocolate (loves your heart)
6. Sea vegetables (full of minerals)
7. Garlic (nature's antibiotic)
8. Avocados (full of good fat)
9. Parsley (the blood cleanser)
10. Wild salmon (keeps your skin young)
11. Beans (lower cholesterol)
12. Kale (powerhouse of nutrients)
13. Green tea (liquid antioxidants)
14. Pumpkin seeds (help the prostate)
15. Microplants (full of nutrients)
16. Oats (the wonder grain)
17. Sweet potatoes (rich in vitamin A)
18. Walnuts (provide essential fatty acids)
19. Yogurt (replants your intestines)
20. Fermented foods (essential digestive aids)

The Familiar and Not-So-Familiar

The majority of these superfoods should not appear unusual; as a matter of fact, most of you probably eat them on a regular basis. Take apples for instance, a favorite snack loaded with antioxidants that can be eaten plain, with a smear of nut butter, or in an apple crumb pie. Blueberries, on any list of favorites, are low in fat and high in fiber and easy to use in smoothies or smothered in another superfood, probiotic-rich yogurt. Perfect for your digestive system, a plain, tart yogurt can be puréed with the powerful cruciferous super vegetable, broccoli, to make a healthy soup or vegetable dip. Quinoa may be new to you, coming only recently to the United States from the mountains of Peru, but its high protein content makes it a must-have on your shopping list. Can't live without chocolate? Go ahead and enjoy a bite of decadence—the darker the healthier.

Land and Sea Vegetables

This superfoods list would not be complete without both land and sea vegetables. The oceans provide an amazing storehouse of mineral-rich foods to rival the most nutrient-dense land produce: dulse, arame, hijiki, and kombu are proving themselves to be effective in weight-loss studies and in preventing osteoporosis. Try pairing them with garlic, known for centuries to be a cure-all for whatever might ail you.

South of the border they know how to appreciate the healthy fats in avocado. These are the "good" fats you want to include in your diet, and when you balance them with a few sprigs of blood-cleansing parsley, everything flows along nicely. Add wild salmon to the menu and you have the ideal source of omega-3 fatty acids, essential fats your body needs for clear beautiful skin, shiny hair, and a well-functioning brain. Beans, a vegetarian source of protein, provide nutrients and fiber. You'll find a wide variety to choose from, including kidney, pinto, cannelli, butter, adzuki, soybeans, black-eyed peas, and lima. Kale is a powerful cancer-fighting vegetable, easy to prepare, and delicious with sautéed garlic.

Rounding Out the Top Twenty

You can sip your antioxidants in green tea and support your prostate and bones with a handful of pumpkin seeds for a snack. If you prefer, add the tea and seeds to a blender with mineral-rich chlorella, spirulina, blue-green algae, or wheat-grass juice, some frozen blueberries, and sweetener of choice for a quick and healthy smoothie.

ESSENTIAL

Wondering what to eat for breakfast? Look no further than a bowl of "the mother of all grains," whole oats cooked overnight in the slow cooker and served warm the next morning with a few tablespoons of walnuts. For lunch, a powerhouse salad of cooked sweet potatoes, high in vitamin A, along with cooked kale, topped with toasted walnuts, and tossed with an apple cider vinaigrette allows for easy digestion and assimilation of nutrients.

Benefits of a Healthy Diet

Eating well optimizes your body's ability to perform. It improves your physical endurance so you can easily handle everyday tasks. Food affects your mental acuity, emotional outlook, personality, and overall sense of well-being, too. A healthy diet provides energy to function optimally, as well as protection from chronic disease.

Specific Health Benefits

A healthy diet will minimize your risk of acquiring many of the chronic diseases currently plaguing our nation. Cardiovascular disease, stroke, diabetes, and certain cancers can all be connected in part to poor diets and failure to maintain healthy weight. Good nutrition improves the overall function of all aspects of the human body, from the way your blood flows to your ability to sleep.

Personal Benefits

On a personal level, taking control of your health through diet is empowering. And if you are in control of your family's diet, the undertaking takes on even greater meaning. There is no better gift you can give your family than the gift of a healthy lifestyle. Developing healthy habits gives them an edge that will last a lifetime.

Healthy Variety

A nutritious diet does not have to be a boring diet. In fact, the healthiest diets are constantly evolving, as you try and add new foods with new combinations of nutrients. Once you have a clear understanding of what your body needs, you'll derive a great deal of pleasure from experimentation and research.

Getting the Kids on Board

Teaching nutrition to kids is easy if you start from scratch, but not everyone has that luxury. Most parents tend to raise their kids as they were raised, and unfortunately not everyone was brought up by nutritionists. Interrupting the sugary soda and crunchy salty snack habits of older kids can be challenging.

When children are small and spend most of their time at home, it is easier to provide only natural, healthy foods. But the minute their care goes into the hands of someone else, be it day care, preschool, or Grandma, health-conscious parents need to go into double-overtime nutrition watch. Once refined sugars and flours are introduced to your child, the battle begins. Sweets are powerful things in the world of child care, and their use as rewards has lifelong implications. To avoid this scenario, insist on maintaining control over your child's diet.

If you are already battling the junk food wars, there are ways to turn the onslaught around. These strategies may take time, but they do work. Bringing kids into the process of planning, shopping, and cooking is the first step.

What's in It for Them?

Just like adults, kids like to see both sides and weigh the good and the bad. Even with young children, "because I said so" is not always effective. You'll get better results if kids can see an upside to the changes you want them to make.

ESSENTIAL

More than 60 percent of children eat too much fat. Less than 20 percent get enough vegetables in their diet. With an average of two trips to the drive-thru each week, it's no wonder. Even so-called "healthy" fast-food choices have hidden fat and sugar in dressings, breads, condiments, sodas, sides, and desserts.

Using outside influences is a great tactic. Find healthy role models for your children. Athletes are obvious choices, but local coaches, dance instructors, and scout leaders also have healthy role model potential. Take a look at your child's activities and start pointing out the healthy active people in their lives.

Finally, give them incentive. It could be having more energy, increased strength for soccer, or better chances at cheerleading tryouts. Both kids and adults need incentive to do new, hard things. It may take some time because for children, unlike adults, a healthy future is not always incentive enough. They do not necessarily see the potential for illness and disease. They are invincible in their own minds, so these goals are less meaningful. Help them find something tangible to work toward that is health- or activity-related. It may require finding them a new hobby or sport, but it's worth the effort. The payoff is a lifelong healthy lifestyle for your children.

Make Kids Part of the Process

Give kids the power of knowledge. Explain the dietary guidelines, and use this knowledge to plan a menu together. Make a shopping list, and take kids with you to the market. Teach them to read the labels and compare nutrients. Give them choices, within parameters, and make them responsible for monitoring their own diets. Most importantly, teach them how to cook. Even very young children can watch and help out in the kitchen, where they'll pick up important knowledge and skills.

From time to time you may need to let actions speak louder than words. A tummy ache can be a powerful tool. Firsthand experience, including real physical results from poor choices, often works better than any incentive or role model. It will give you both a reference point from which to continue the work of daily nutrition.

Most importantly, as a parent, you must never give in. Regardless of how much control you allow kids, you are still in charge. Don't slip into the fast-and-easy. It is your job to show them what a healthy lifestyle is. Being strict and vigilant in the early years will pay off with healthy active teens and adults.

Small Changes Can Lead to Huge Successes

The stress of trying to get your child to eat makes mealtime difficult for the child as well as the parent. The goal is to make every meal an adventure instead of a battle, which sometimes requires thinking outside of the box. Think creatively or even like a child, and eventually mealtime will become fun and enjoyable again.

Remember the ABCs to restricted eaters:

- Avoid letting your child think, "if I don't like it, Mom or Dad will make me something different."

- Be consistent with the guidelines you choose to put in place.
- Construct a positive, calm environment during mealtimes.

The "I Don't Like It" Protocol:

- Start small. Try putting new things on your child's plate, even if it's just five peas.
- If kids try X, Y, and Z, then they can have something they like.
- However, don't make the mistake of giving them their absolute favorite food. For example, if they like peanut butter and jelly, but love chicken nuggets, give them the PB & J.
- Make sure you're only cooking one dinner for the family. You didn't open a catering service. You should be satisfied that you are providing a complete nutritious meal that will promote health and growth.
- If food items are not tried, place the meal in refrigerator. Offer the meal one last time around 7:00 P.M., before bedtime. Don't cook a new meal. Missing one meal will not cause kids any harm—they will be fine until breakfast.
- Focus on one meal. The best meal to focus on is usually dinner. You don't have to implement new rules every night at the beginning. Gradually work in these rules/behavior changes on specific nights.
- Have your child sign a contract to promise to try the new foods you introduce (at least one full bite).
- As a general rule, you have to try a food fifteen times before your mouth decides if it likes it or not. So, give it a chance.

The Ideal Pantry

An ideal pantry should be well organized, enabling you to easily choose a lean protein, a fiber source, and flavorful ingredients in a matter of two minutes to put together a delicious, complete meal. The first step in setting up an efficient pantry is taking a trip to the grocery store, farmer's market, and so on. You may refer to the information in Chapter 17 to ensure your list is nutritionally complete. If your shopping list is balanced, your shopping cart will be balanced, and your pantry will be balanced.

Be prepared for those days of last-minute ordeals that can cause your routine or plan to go astray. Make sure to have a variety of frozen vegetables, cans of beans, quick-cooking grains such as couscous, and frozen entrées such as Kashi, Lean Cuisine, and Amy's Organic on hand. Then, if necessary, preparing a meal in minutes becomes relatively easy. You could simply heat an entire frozen bag of vegetables and a frozen entrée to have a complete meal ready in minutes. Keep other proteins available such as frozen shrimp, individual chicken breasts, turkey burgers, chicken sausages, fish fillets, and marinated tofu.

Each pantry should contain whole grains such as quinoa, whole-wheat couscous, millet, bulgur, brown rice, whole-grain breads, cereals, and whole-wheat pasta. Because foods come packaged in a variety of ways it is often difficult to accurately define the correct portion. You may want to create a snack basket with snack baggies filled with the appropriate portions of oat bran pretzels, nuts, soy crisps, and so on.

Be sure to keep measuring cups handy to scoop cereals and other grains. It's always a great idea to use measuring cups as serving utensils, so you know how much you're eating. Proteins can be measured with a small kitchen scale to monitor portion sizes. Personal preferences can create chaos in pantries if communication is not practiced. If there are specific nutritional needs or preferences among household members, be sure there are designated areas for these specific food choices.

CHAPTER 3

The Power of Protein

Protein is one of the macronutrients and most important sources of calories to be consumed at each meal, including snacks. Its power to slow digestion and regulate blood sugars, hunger, and energy levels can improve your productivity and performance—and you won't need to take so many coffee breaks. This is especially true during that afternoon drop, when many of us reach for a quick fix of processed foods or "empty calories." Luckily, we have plenty of protein sources from plants, animals, and dairy products to save us from malnutrition and help us reach our potential.

The Role of Protein in a Healthy Diet

Protein builds and maintains muscles, organs, connective tissues, skin, bones, teeth, blood, and your DNA (deoxyribonucleic acid). It helps the body heal when it is sick, wounded, or depleted. Without protein, even mild exercise would weaken you to the point of exhaustion.

Protein contributes to the formation of enzymes. Almost all reactions that occur in the body, such as digestion, require enzymes. Enzymes are catalysts to these reactions, increasing the rate at which they occur.

There is protein in your blood, called antibodies. They serve as your body's immune responders. They bind with and fight foreign invaders, such as bacteria or toxins. Protein is found in hormones, your body's chemical messengers. Hormones help regulate the body's activities, maintaining balance or homeostasis.

Amino Acids

Protein is composed of twenty amino acids. These acids link together in chains to form the variety of proteins your body needs. The length and shape of the chain determines the protein's structure. Of the twenty amino acids, eleven of them are made by your body. These eleven acids are called nonessential because you do not need to consume them. The remaining nine amino acids are called essential, and it is important that you eat these every day. Getting all nine essential amino acids is not hard, especially if you eat meat. Animal foods (which include meat, eggs, and dairy products) contain the largest concentration of protein. Animal protein is considered complete, because it contains all nine essential amino acids.

ESSENTIAL

Eating complementary protein means consuming both beans and grains every day. The beans can be pinto, kidney, black, lentils, garbanzo, split peas, or peanuts. Grains should be whole, including brown rice, whole-wheat pasta, bread, crackers, or tortillas. Sesame seeds also complement the protein of beans.

Plant foods also contain proteins, but few plants contain complete protein. This is one of the challenges of vegetarianism, because to stay healthy you must consume enough foods with the right mixture of amino acids. It sounds complicated, but grains, nuts, and legumes contain the proteins that are not found in other plants, so adding a variety of these to your diet does the trick.

Plant foods eaten in combination to create complete protein are called complementary proteins. When these foods are eaten over the course of a day, protein intake is complete. Protein derived from complementary plant proteins is considered a healthy alternative, and by many people, a superior one. Eating such combinations of plant foods not only completes the protein, but also provides other nutrients vital to good health as well, most notably fiber, vitamins, and minerals. And most plants do all that without saturated fat.

Cooking Protein

Cooked protein is also referred to as denatured. When denatured, protein changes its structure and stops functioning. In denaturation, the amino acids loosen, recoil, and tighten, which changes the appearance, texture, and flavor of the protein. If you watch an egg being cooked, you can see the denaturation happen within a minute or two as the albumen turns white.

Cooking protein does not necessarily require heat. Acid will denature protein, as it does in the Latin American dish ceviche, in which seafood is marinated in lime. Salt is used to cook protein in cured meats, such as ham, sausages, and salt cod. Pickled meats combine acid and salt for a double-whammy cooking method. Even agitation can denature protein, as in the whipping of eggs. In this case prolonged agitation changes the egg's structure, making it safe to eat. Meringue demonstrates this effect on the egg white, while yolks and whole eggs get this treatment in mayonnaise and emulsified salad dressings, such as those used in Caesar salad.

FACT

Denaturation of protein doesn't happen only in the kitchen. You saw it during your last visit to the beach. The waves break onto the sand, the tide rolls in and out, and that motion denatures the proteins in the seawater, creating sea foam.

Choosing Your Protein

People in the United States overconsume animal protein. To stay healthy and rebuild muscle, the average adult needs only five to six ounces of complete protein each day. But a typical American diet consists of bacon and eggs for breakfast, a meat-filled sandwich for lunch, and a dinner featuring meat as its focus. A healthy family needs a healthy diet of lean protein in moderation. Animal proteins are higher in fat, particularly saturated fat, which in turn makes them high in cholesterol. Plant foods, however, contain no cholesterol, less fat (in the form of plant oil), and lots of fiber.

Eating too little protein is not healthy, but neither is eating too much. Overeating protein does not build extra muscle. The protein your body does not utilize is stored as fat.

Meat

Meat is a common generic term meaning flesh, but to chefs it refers specifically to the flesh of four-legged domesticated animals. This includes mainly beef, lamb, and pork. Lamb is becoming popular in America, and pork is gaining in popularity as a lean meat option. But by far, the favorite meat in the United States is beef.

Historically, the cow's size made it more valuable as a draft animal than a source of food. The logistics of slaughtering such a large animal were daunting. Salting was the main method of preserving meat, and this method was not very sophisticated. So, unless there was a real crowd to feed, lamb was a more popular choice. But modern Americans love what cows offer. The cow's meat, milk, and hide easily make it the world's most important domesticated animal.

Choosing Beef

Beef and veal are readily available in modern supermarkets, and for the most part, quality is high. The United States Department of Agriculture (USDA) grades meat for consumption based on muscle-to-bone and fat-to-muscle ratios. Beef grades, from best to worse, are prime, choice, and select. Lesser grades, used mainly for processed meat products, include standard, commercial, and utility. Grades are stamped in purple on the outer carcass of the animal, and are usually prominently advertised by retailers, especially when the grade is high.

Beef cows are taken to market when they are between eighteen and twenty-four months of age. Before that time the cow is considered veal. Veal is a male dairy cow between sixteen and eighteen months of age. Veal grades, from best to worse, are prime, choice, good, standard, and utility.

The Disadvantages of Meat

Meat is generally considered a high-fat protein choice. Usually fat means flavor. In today's world people appreciate, and even expect, a high level of flavor in their meat, despite full knowledge that saturated fat contributes to coronary artery disease and elevated cholesterol levels.

Lean cuts are available, but even if you cannot see the fat marbled throughout a particular cut, the saturated fat is still present within the muscle cells. When meat is heated, the fat melts and penetrates the muscle. So even if you do not eat the visible fat on a steak, you are consuming saturated fat.

This appetite for fatty beef has drastically changed the landscape of modern agriculture. Today cattle are bred and raised to provide the most meat with the least cost. According to the USDA, the average American consumes sixty-seven pounds of beef every year.

A wild cow would naturally consume fiber-rich plants that are unsuitable for human consumption. Today, cows compete with humans for food, consuming grain grown on valuable fertile soil. In the United States, half of the water and 80 percent of the grain harvested goes to feed livestock.

Poultry

Poultry is a term used to describe domesticated birds raised for food. In the United States this means mainly chicken and turkey. Game hens are another form of poultry that can be found in some supermarkets. Duck, although common in Europe and Asia, appears more often on restaurant menus than in your average American grocery store.

Most supermarkets offer organic, free-range, and natural birds. Free-range chickens have more flavor because they are allowed to exercise a bit more. Natural birds contain nothing synthetic, no preservatives or artificial flavoring or colorings, but standards permit antibiotics and hormone use. Organic birds are fed grains that have not been exposed to chemicals and pesticides. They may not be treated with antibiotics or drugs, and must be allowed to go outside and exercise.

ALERT

Whenever possible, buy free-range, organic poultry. Common chickens are raised with profit, not health, in mind. They must be fed antibiotics to fend off disease. They are given growth hormones, which, coupled with lack of exercise, makes them so fat they cannot move. In addition, the food they are fed is grown with artificial fertilizers and chemical pesticides.

Kosher chickens are organic and free-range, and are processed under the strict supervision of a rabbi. They are also soaked in salty brine, which gives them a unique flavor.

When shopping for chickens, frugal cooks know that whole chickens are always less expensive than cut-up parts. But unless you possess good butchering skills, it can be worth paying a little more. Keep in mind that chicken fat occurs in and around the skin, which is easy to remove.

Seafood

Seafood is the most abundant source of protein on earth. Consider all the varieties, around the world, and it's an immense category of food. Narrowed down to its basic parts, the world of seafood is easy to navigate. Seafood is a name given to all marine animals caught or raised for food. This includes both fresh and saltwater species. People tend to condense them all into a general category of fish, but there are many subcategories.

Fish Groups

Fish is first divided into two basic types: finfish and shellfish. There are two kinds of finfish: flat fish and round fish. The flat fish, which include flounder, halibut, and sole, skim along the bottom of the sea. Round fish (which only appear round if they are swimming straight toward you) are found in both freshwater and saltwater. Freshwater fish have much smaller bones than their larger, oceangoing cousins. Shellfish are also separated into two categories: mollusks, such as mussels and clams, and crustaceans, which include crabs, lobsters, crayfish, and shrimp.

Choosing Fish

If you are lucky enough to live near the sea, you will likely have an abundance of fish at your market. Further inland, your fish selection may be more limited. Luckily, frozen fish today are of very high quality, as they are flash-frozen on board the ship that caught them.

When buying frozen fish, be sure it is free of ice, which is a sign that it has been defrosted and refrozen. The fish should have a natural shape, with only a light coating of frost. Defrost frozen fish slowly, twenty-four to thirty-six hours in the refrigerator is best. Place defrosting fish in a colander or perforated pan to separate the runoff juices. Smaller pieces can be cooked frozen.

When buying fresh fish, be sure that all you smell is fresh, oceany fish. If the smell is off-putting, don't buy it. When you get the fish home, store it in the fridge loosely covered with paper, preferably in a perforated pan to allow juices to drain away. If you plan to store the fish longer than two to three days, it should be frozen.

Eggs

The nutritional value of eggs cannot be denied. They are loaded with protein and are, as such, used as a measure for other proteins. What's more, they contain almost every essential vitamin and mineral humans need.

Egg yolks contain a high percentage of cholesterol, and people watching their cholesterol should avoid them. But normal, healthy, active humans can, and should, benefit from the incredible egg.

Choosing Your Eggs

When possible, look for organic eggs from free-range chickens. They are regulated to a certain extent by the USDA. No antibiotics or hormones are allowed, and the birds are provided with access to the outdoors. Eggs have a tremendous shelf life. By the time they get to your grocer, they are usually one or two weeks old. They will last in your fridge another three weeks. The shell, which is very porous, allows odor and moisture to pass through. Over time, the yolk and white become thinner. Thicker, fresher egg whites and yolks are preferable for recipes that require the eggs to be whipped.

Beans

The general term *bean* encompasses several plants and usually refers to the legume, a large plant seed found within long pods from the plant family Fabaceae. Soybeans, peas, lentils, and kidney beans are examples of legumes. When the seeds are dried, they are referred to as pulses. Many beans are only sold in dry form, although some, such as the pea, come both dried and fresh.

Beans are an excellent source of low-fat protein, containing more than twice the amount of protein as grain. You can buy beans in dried or canned form. Dried beans take longer to cook, and must first undergo a long soaking process to tenderize them. Canned beans are readily available, which makes it easy to add beans into your everyday diet. Most supermarkets stock such common beans as adzuki, black, broad bean, cannellini, chickpeas, fava, garbanzo, kidney, lentil, lima, mung, navy, pea, pinto, runner, soy, and white.

Nuts

Botanically, a nut is a fruit with one seed. The wall of the seed becomes very hard, and the meat of the seed stays very loose within. Walnuts, pecans, hazelnuts, and chestnuts fall into this category. However, in the world of cuisine there are other nuts that do not fit the definition. Peanuts are legumes, the pine nut is a seed from a pine tree, a macadamia nut is a kernel, and the Brazil nut is found inside a fruit capsule.

Nuts have a high oil content and can easily become rancid if stored improperly. Heat and light increase rancidity, so refrigeration is best for long-term storage. Flavor is greatly altered, and generally improved, by heat. Toasting nuts in an oven yields the best results. Spread them out on a baking sheet and roast at 350°F for 10–15 minutes, until they become fragrant.

Recipes

Lemon Sesame Tuna

Tuna is delicious as an appetizer when it's cut into cubes and marinated in a lemon mixture.

INGREDIENTS | SERVES 8

2 tablespoons lemon juice

1 tablespoon low-sodium soy sauce

1 tablespoon sesame oil

2 green onions, minced

2 (⅓-pound) tuna filets

¼ cup sesame seeds, toasted

1. In shallow bowl, combine lemon juice, soy sauce, sesame oil, and green onions and mix well. Cut the tuna into 1" cubes and add to the marinade; toss to coat and let stand for 15 minutes.

2. Preheat oven to 400°F. Arrange the fish in a single layer on a baking sheet. Bake until fish is just opaque, about 5–7 minutes. Sprinkle with sesame seeds and serve immediately with toothpicks.

PER SERVING Calories: 73 • Fat: 4.8 g • Protein: 6.6 g • Sodium: 78 mg • Carbohydrates: 1.2 g • Fiber: 0.65 g

Poached Chicken with Pears and Herbs

Pears pair well with all poultry. Try this dish for a quick dinner or double the recipe for company.

INGREDIENTS | SERVES 2

1 ripe pear, peeled, cored, and cut in chunks

2 shallots, minced

½ cup dry white wine

1 teaspoon rosemary, dried, or 1 tablespoon fresh

1 teaspoon thyme, dried, or 1 tablespoon fresh

2½ pounds chicken breasts, boneless and skinless

Salt and pepper, to taste

Prepare the poaching liquid by mixing the first five ingredients and bringing to a boil in a saucepan. Season the chicken with salt and pepper and add to the pan. Simmer slowly for 10 minutes. Serve with pears on top of each piece.

PER SERVING Calories: 307 • Fat: 9 g • Protein: 41 g • Sodium: 2 mg • Carbohydrates: 15 g • Fiber: 2 g

Gingered Tofu and Bok Choy Stir-Fry

Dark, leafy bok choy is a highly nutritious vegetable that can be found in well-stocked groceries. Keep an eye out for light-green baby bok choy, which is a bit more tender but carries a similar flavor.

INGREDIENTS | SERVES 3

3 tablespoons soy sauce

2 tablespoons lemon or lime juice

1 tablespoon fresh ginger, minced

1 block firm or extra-firm tofu, well pressed

2 tablespoons olive oil

1 head bok choy or 3–4 small baby bok choys

½ teaspoon sugar

½ teaspoon sesame oil

1. Whisk together soy sauce, lemon or lime juice, and ginger in a shallow pan. Cut tofu into cubes, and marinate for at least 1 hour. Drain, reserving marinade.

2. In a large skillet, sauté tofu in olive oil for 3–4 minutes.

3. Stir in reserved marinade, bok choy, and sugar.

4. Cook, stirring, for 3–4 more minutes, or until bok choy is done.

5. Drizzle with sesame oil and serve over rice.

PER SERVING Calories: 243 • Fat: 18 g • Protein: 19 g • Sodium: 732 mg • Carbohydrates: 8 g • Fiber: 4 g

Crab Cakes with Sesame Crust

Remember to pick through the crabmeat and remove any cartilage or bits of shell that can be left behind during processing.

INGREDIENTS | SERVES 5

1 pound (16 ounces) lump crabmeat

1 egg

1 tablespoon minced fresh ginger

1 small scallion, finely chopped

1 tablespoon dry sherry

1 tablespoon freshly squeezed lemon juice

6 tablespoons mayonnaise

Sea salt and freshly ground white pepper to taste (optional)

Old Bay Seasoning to taste (optional)

¼ cup lightly toasted sesame seeds

1. Preheat oven to 375°F. In a large bowl, mix together the crab, egg, ginger, scallion, sherry, lemon juice, mayonnaise, and the seasonings, if using.

2. Form the mixture into 10 equal cakes. Spread the sesame seeds over a sheet pan and dip both sides of the cakes to coat them. Arrange the crab cakes on a baking sheet treated with nonstick spray. Typical baking time is 8–10 minutes (depending on how thick you make the cakes).

PER SERVING Calories: 107.69 • Fat: 6.45 g • Protein: 9.04 g • Sodium: 170.88 mg • Carbohydrate: 2.93 g • Fiber: 0.60 g

Salmon Cakes with Mango Salsa

If you cannot find almond or pecan meal, you can make your own by grinding a cup of raw almonds or pecans in a food processor until a flour consistency is achieved. Be careful not to grind them so long they become an oily paste.

INGREDIENTS | SERVES 4

1 (14-ounce) can wild Alaskan salmon
¼ cup minced chives
1 large egg, beaten
1 cup almond or pecan flour
Sea salt, to taste
1 ripe mango
½ red bell pepper
½ sweet Vidalia onion
3-inch piece gingerroot
Juice of 1 lemon

Grilled Salmon and Salsa

A beautiful fillet of grilled salmon would benefit from a few tablespoons of mango or tomato salsa. The juices will enrich the dry meat, and the sweet-sour taste will complement the smoky flavor of the fish. Serve alongside some steamed broccoli tossed with garlic sautéed in olive oil and a salad of cooked kale and walnuts. A true superfood!

1. Preheat oven to 350°F.

2. In a medium bowl, combine salmon, chives, beaten egg, nut flour, and sea salt.

3. Mix well; form into 4 patties.

4. Place on a well-oiled baking sheet; bake 15–20 minutes, or cook in an oiled skillet, browning on both sides.

5. To make the salsa, peel and chop mango into small pieces; place in a medium-size bowl.

6. Mince red pepper and onion; add to bowl.

7. Peel and grate ginger, extracting juice by pressing the fiber against the side of a shallow dish; pour juice into bowl with mango mixture.

8. Juice the lemon; add to mango mixture; mix well.

9. Cover and refrigerate until ready to serve. For a hotter, spicier version, add a fresh, minced jalapeño pepper.

PER SERVING Calories: 260 • Fat: 8 g • Protein: 30 g • Sodium: 52 mg • Carbohydrates: 18 g • Fiber: 4 g

Grilled Fish and Spinach Packets

This beautiful method of cooking delicate fish is perfect for entertaining. The packets make a gorgeous presentation.

INGREDIENTS | SERVES 4

1 tablespoon olive oil
1 onion, chopped
2 cloves garlic, minced
¼ cup dry white wine
¼ teaspoon salt
⅛ teaspoon white pepper
1 tablespoon chopped fresh tarragon
1 (10-ounce) package fresh baby spinach
1 pound fish fillets, of your choice
1 green bell pepper, julienned

En Papillote

Food cooked in foil or parchment paper is called *en papillote*. This method of cooking keeps food moist—it's an excellent way to cook delicate foods such as greens and fish. The food steams in the packet, sealing in juices and flavor. Warn your guests to be careful opening these packets because steam will billow out.

1. Prepare and preheat grill. In a small skillet, heat oil over medium heat. Add onion and garlic; cook and stir until tender, about 6–7 minutes. Remove from heat and stir in wine, salt, and pepper.

2. Return to high heat and boil until reduced by half, about 5 minutes. Remove from heat and stir in tarragon. Set aside.

3. Tear off four 12" × 18" pieces of heav-duty foil and place on work surface. Divide spinach into quarters and place on foil. Cut fish into four pieces and place on top of spinach. Spoon onion mixture on fish and top with green bell pepper strips.

4. Bring up long edges of foil and, leaving some space for steam expansion, seal with a double fold, then fold in short ends to seal. Place on grill rack 6 inches from medium coals. Grill, turning packets twice and rearranging on grill, until fish flakes easily when tested with fork, about 15–20 minutes. Serve immediately.

PER SERVING Calories: 171.73 • Fat: 4.55 grams • Protein: 18 g • Sodium: 286.52 mg • Carbohydrates: 2 g • Fiber: 1g

Asian-Style Fish Cakes

TIP: For crunchy fish cakes, coat each side in the rice flour, and then lightly spritz the top of the patties with olive or peanut oil before baking as directed.

INGREDIENTS | SERVES 8

1 pound catfish fillets

2 green onions, minced

1 banana pepper, cored, seeded, and chopped

2 cloves garlic, minced

1 tablespoon grated or minced ginger

1 tablespoon Bragg's Liquid Aminos

1 tablespoon lemon juice

1 teaspoon lemon zest

Optional seasonings to taste:

Old Bay Seasoning

Rice flour

Olive or peanut oil

1. Preheat oven to 375°F. Cut the fish into 1-inch pieces and combine with the green onions, banana pepper, garlic, ginger, Bragg's Liquid Aminos, lemon juice, and lemon zest in a food processor. Process until chopped and mixed. (You do not want to purée this mixture; it should be a rough chop.) Add the Old Bay Seasoning, if using, and stir to mix.

2. Form the fish mixture into patties of about 2 tablespoons each; you should have 16 patties total. Place the patties on a baking sheet treated with nonstick cooking spray, and bake for 12–15 minutes, or until crisp. (Alternatively, you can fry these in a nonstick pan for about 4 minutes on each side.)

PER SERVING Calories: 65.98 • Fat: 1.66 g • Protein: 11.02 g • Sodium: 112.44 mg • Carbohydrate: 1.22 g • Fiber: 0.36 mg

Not All Weeds Are Bad

Seaweed is an important ingredient in many processed foods, such as commercial ice cream and other foods that contain carrageenan, a thickener found in several kinds of seaweed.

Venison with Dried Cranberry Vinegar Sauce

Mild-tasting farm-raised venison is available at many supermarkets and meat markets.

INGREDIENTS | SERVES 4

⅛ cup (2 tablespoons) dried cranberries

1 tablespoon sugar

3 tablespoons water

⅛ cup (2 tablespoons) champagne or white wine vinegar

2 teaspoons olive oil

1 tablespoon minced shallots or red onion

1 teaspoon minced garlic

⅛ cup (2 tablespoons) dry red wine

½ cup low-fat, reduced-sodium chicken broth

½ teaspoon cracked black pepper

½ pound (8 ounces) cooked venison

1 teaspoon cornstarch or potato flour

2 teaspoons butter

Operate Your Appliances Safely

When puréeing hot mixtures, leave the vent uncovered on your food processor. If you're using a blender, either remove the vent cover from the lid or leave the lid ajar so the steam can escape.

1. Add the cranberries, sugar, water, and champagne (or vinegar) to a saucepan, and bring to a boil. Reduce the heat and simmer for 5 minutes. Remove from heat and transfer to a food processor or blender; process until the cranberries are chopped; it isn't necessary to purée because you want some cranberry "chunks" to remain. Set aside.

2. Pour the olive oil into a heated nonstick skillet; add the shallots and garlic, and sauté for 30 seconds. Deglaze the pan with the red wine, and cook, stirring occasionally, until the wine is reduced by half. Add the cranberry mixture and the chicken broth, and bring to a boil. Reduce the heat to medium low, season with the pepper, add the venison, and simmer for 3 minutes, or until the meat is heated through.

3. Thicken the sauce, using a slurry of cornstarch or potato flour and 1 tablespoon of water; simmer until the sauce thickens. You'll need to cook the sauce a bit longer if you use cornstarch in order to remove the "starchy" taste. Remove from the heat, add the butter, and whisk to incorporate the butter into the sauce.

PER SERVING (WITHOUT CORNSTARCH OR FLOUR) Calories: 154.14 • Fat: 6.05 g • Protein: 17.48 g • Sodium: 76.56 mg • Carbohydrate: 4.36 g • Fiber: 0.07 g

Beautiful Black-Eyed Pea Burgers

Rich in iron, calcium, and vitamin A, black-eyed peas add nutrition as well as strong meaty flavor to soups and vegan burgers.

INGREDIENTS | SERVES 6

1 cup black-eyed peas, soaked
Spring water, as needed
1 stamp-sized piece kombu, soaked
1 tablespoon umeboshi paste
2 medium scallions, chopped
¼ cup safflower oil

1. Rinse beans and place in pressure cooker. Add enough water to cover beans. Bring to boil. Skim off foam. Add kombu. Cover, bring to pressure, lower heat, and pressure cook for 20 minutes (or simmer on stove 1 hour).

2. Mash beans. Season with umeboshi paste. Add scallions.

3. Form bean purée into 6–8 patties. Place in refrigerator to firm. In a skillet, pan fry patties in oil until browned on both sides.

PER SERVING Calories: 107 • Fat: 9 g • Protein: 1 g • Sodium: 187 mg • Carbohydrate: 5 g • Fiber: 2 g

Moroccan Lamb Stew

Look for boneless, lean lamb chops to dice for this recipe; it is cheaper and easier than buying a whole leg of lamb.

INGREDIENTS | SERVES 2

½ pound lean boneless lamb, cubed
2 cloves garlic, minced
½ onion, chopped
2 tablespoons lemon juice
¼ cup sliced green olives
2 teaspoons honey
¼ teaspoon salt
½ teaspoon freshly ground black pepper
¼ teaspoon turmeric
2 sprigs fresh thyme

Place the lamb, garlic, onion, lemon juice, olives, honey, salt, pepper, and turmeric in a 2-quart slow cooker. Top with the sprigs of thyme. Cook on low for 8 hours.

PER SERVING Calories: 280 • Fat: 11 g • Protein: 32 g • Sodium: 630 mg • Carbohydrates: 13 g • Fiber: 2 g

Salmon with Lemon, Capers, and Rosemary

Salmon is amazingly moist and tender when cooked in a slow cooker.

INGREDIENTS | SERVES 2

8 ounces salmon

⅓ cup water

2 tablespoons lemon juice

3 thin slices fresh lemon

1 tablespoon nonpareil capers

½ teaspoon minced fresh rosemary

1. Place the salmon on the bottom of a 2-quart slow cooker. Pour the water and lemon juice over the fish. Arrange the lemon slices in a single layer on top of the fish. Sprinkle with capers and rosemary.

2. Cook on low for 2 hours. Discard lemon slices prior to serving.

PER SERVING Calories: 170 • Fat: 7 g • Protein: 23 g • Sodium: 180 mg • Carbohydrates: 2 g • Fiber: 0 g

Hawaiian-Style Mahi-Mahi

The fish is gently poached in a tasty liquid, which infuses it with flavor.

INGREDIENTS | SERVES 6

6 (4-ounce) mahi-mahi fillets

12 ounces pineapple juice

3 tablespoons grated fresh ginger

¼ cup lime juice

3 tablespoons ponzu sauce

1. Place the fillets in a 6-quart slow cooker. Top with the remaining ingredients. Cook on low for 5 hours or until the fish is fully cooked.

2. Remove the fillets and discard the cooking liquid.

PER SERVING Calories: 140 • Fat: 1 g • Protein: 21 g • Sodium: 100 mg • Carbohydrates: 10 g • Fiber: 0 g

Balsamic Chicken and Spinach

Serve this with rice pilaf.

INGREDIENTS | SERVES 4

¾ pound boneless, skinless chicken breasts, cut into strips

¼ cup balsamic vinegar

4 cloves garlic, minced

1 tablespoon minced fresh oregano

1 tablespoon minced fresh Italian parsley

½ teaspoon freshly ground black pepper

5 ounces baby spinach

1. Place the chicken, vinegar, garlic, and spices into a 4-quart slow cooker. Stir. Cook on low for 6 hours.

2. Stir in the baby spinach and continue to cook until it starts to wilt, about 15 minutes. Stir before serving.

PER SERVING Calories: 180 • Fat: 3 g • Protein: 28 g • Sodium: 125 mg • Carbohydrates: 10 g • Fiber: 2 g

Mango Duck Breast

Slow-cooked mangoes soften and create their own sauce in this easy duck dish.

INGREDIENTS | SERVES 4

2 boneless, skinless duck breasts

1 large mango, cubed

¼ cup duck or chicken stock

1 tablespoon ginger juice

1 tablespoon minced hot pepper

1 tablespoon minced shallot

Place all ingredients into a 4-quart slow cooker. Cook on low for 4 hours.

PER SERVING Calories: 150 • Fat: 4 g • Protein: 17 g • Sodium: 70 mg • Carbohydrates: 10 g • Fiber: 1 g

Raw Sushi Nori Rolls

These nori rolls are delicious dipped into nama shoyu sauce and wasabi or homemade horseradish sauce, and are wonderful paired with miso soup.

INGREDIENTS | SERVES 2

2 sheets raw or roasted nori

¼ cup Almond Garlic Pâté (included in this chapter) for each sheet

4 tablespoons microgreen sprouts (alfalfa, sunflower, clover, or radish) per sheet

2 tablespoons, or more, finely grated carrot per sheet

½ avocado, sliced

Nori

Nori is a nutritious sea vegetable high in minerals and vitamins that is prepared in thin sheets. Nori is used as the wrap for sushi, and the texture makes a perfect replacement for tortilla wraps. Like other sea veggies, nori is high in iodine content, as well as iron, calcium, vitamins A, B, and C, and carotene.

1. Lay 1 nori sheet flat on a sushi mat. Spread about ¼ cup of the pâté across one end of the nori. Add a layer of sprouts and top with the carrot and avocado.

2. Roll up the nori sheets tightly using a sushi mat. Just before completing the roll, dip your finger in water and run it along the edge of the nori sheet to create a seal.

3. Cut the sushi rolls into 6 round pieces with a sharp knife (ideally one with saw teeth) using a gentle seesaw motion. Repeat the process with the remaining nori sheet.

PER SERVING Calories: 194 • Fat: 16 g • Protein: 6 g • Sodium: 312 mg • Carbohydrates: 8 g • Fiber: 6 g

Almond Garlic Pâté

This is a recipe for a basic raw pâté. You may substitute other nuts and seeds to vary the flavor. This recipe has many uses: as a spread on crackers or flatbread, a dip for celery sticks, or a filling in nori rolls, burritos, or wraps.

INGREDIENTS | SERVES 2–4

2 cups almonds, soaked

1 cup cashews, soaked but crispy

¼ cup celery hearts or fennel bulb, chopped

4 tablespoons red or white onion, or scallions, chopped

2 tablespoons lemon juice

2 cloves garlic

¼ teaspoon salt

1. Soak the almonds and sunflower seeds in water for 8 to 12 hours.

2. Blend all the ingredients together in a food processor using the S blade, or homogenize it using a heavy-duty juicer.

PER SERVING Calories: 521 • Fat: 44 g • Protein: 19 g • Sodium: 151 mg • Carbohydrates: 109.4 g • Fiber: 11 g

Pâté

This is high-protein staple on a raw foods diet. This basic pâté will stay fresh for about a week in the refrigerator because the salt and lemon juice help preserve it. You can take the pâté to work with a salad for a quick and satisfying lunch. When you are ready to use the pâté, take out 1 cup and keep the rest in the refrigerator. Mix 1 cup of the pâté mix with your favorite spices for a different flavor at each meal.

CHAPTER 4

The Importance of Carbohydrates

Carbohydrates are necessary for achieving optimal health, and are found in four of the major food groups: whole grains, fruit, vegetables, and dairy products. These are your body and brain's main source of fuel. Carbohydrates are also needed to maintain proper function of the central nervous system, muscles, and metabolism of fat and protein. Today, we find carbohydrates in many forms, making it difficult to distinguish which ones are truly beneficial for us. All carbohydrates break down into sugar in your blood, which causes your pancreas to release insulin that transports sugar to your cells for energy. However, the rate at which food breaks down into sugar determines if your energy levels are going to be stable or climb quickly then crash. Fiber found in carbohydrates slows digestion and helps keep energy levels and hunger in check.

Simple Carbohydrates

Simple carbohydrates are the sugars. They are grouped by the number of molecules from which they are made. Single sugars, or monosaccharides, have one molecule. They include glucose, fructose, and galactose. Sugars composed of two molecules are called disaccharides. They include lactose, maltose, sucrose, and honey.

Glucose

Glucose is made by plants during photosynthesis as energy for the plant. Glucose is found in plants, fruits, and honey. Also known as dextrose, it is the human body's first source of energy. Most of the carbohydrates you eat are broken down into glucose by the body. Glucose is absorbed directly into the bloodstream, concentrating in the blood. This concentration is measured as your blood sugar level. You must eat 50 to 100 grams of carbohydrates each day to maintain good blood sugar levels.

Fructose and Galactose

Fructose is also found in honey, fruits, and plants. It is sweeter than glucose and table sugar. Galactose occurs in nature only as one of the two molecules that make up lactose.

Lactose

Also known as milk sugar, lactose is a disaccharide composed of one glucose and one galactose molecule. Found naturally in milk, it is the only animal-based carbohydrate. It is not commonly thought of as a sugar because it is not nearly as sweet as glucose.

Maltose

This disaccharide is composed of two glucose molecules. It is mainly seen in sprouting grains and is a vital component of beer. Brewers soak grain, usually barley, in water, until germination. The maltose is also extracted and used to make malt syrup, a common ingredient in artisan breads.

Refined Sugar: Sucrose

Sucrose is ordinary table sugar, derived from sugar cane and sugar beets. It is composed of one glucose and one fructose molecule. It occurs in small amounts in most fruits and is the most widely used sweetener in American homes. Sucrose provides quick energy, but it is stripped of its additional nutrients in the refining process, so it is not the ideal form of carbohydrate. The human body needs the entire natural package of a piece of fruit, or a tablespoon of honey, which, unlike table sugar, also includes fiber, water, vitamins, and minerals. For more on refined sugar, and ways to sweeten your day without it, see Chapter 6.

Honey

This disaccharide is also composed of one glucose and one fructose molecule. Honey is more concentrated than sucrose, which makes it twice as sweet. Consequently, less is needed when it's used as a sweetener. The body breaks down and uses both sucrose and honey in the same way, but honey is a naturally occurring sweetener that needs no refinement. It contains other elements that are considered healthful, including vitamins, minerals, fiber, and antioxidants. Honey can be substituted for granulated sugar as a sweetener, but because it is twice as sweet, use half as much.

Complex Carbohydrates

Complex carbohydrates are found in plant foods that contain starch and fiber. They are known as polysaccharides, meaning more than two sugars. They come in chains of thousands of glucose molecules. In order to be absorbed, your body must break apart these molecule chains. It takes considerably more effort for your body to absorb polysaccharides than it does to absorb single or double sugars.

Starch is found in grains, root vegetables, nuts, seeds, and fruits. It can gelatinize, meaning that it gets thick and absorbs water when heated.

Fiber, mainly found in plant cell walls, comes in two varieties: water-soluble and water-insoluble. Both types of fiber are essential for good health.

Water-soluble fiber includes substances such as pectin. When water is added, this fiber absorbs it like a sponge and swells. This type of fiber seems to help lower blood cholesterol levels, especially in conjunction with a diet low in fat. It also tends to delay the emptying of the stomach, so food is absorbed more slowly, causing that full feeling to last longer. Water-soluble fiber is found in beans, some grains including oats and barley, and fruits and vegetables such as apples and carrots.

Water-insoluble fiber, which includes cellulose, doesn't swell nearly as much as water-soluble fiber. This is found in the structural parts of the plant—skin, seeds, and stems. Bran and any whole grain that still includes its outer hull, such as brown rice, are great sources of insoluble fiber.

Unlike starch, fiber-based polysaccharides cannot be broken apart by our digestive enzymes. This fiber keeps waste moving through the intestines, which helps prevent disorders of the lower intestine. Complex carbohydrates are thought to play a role in the prevention of colon cancer by reducing the amount of time cancer-causing agents spend in the intestine.

Refined Flour

White flour is a commonly consumed starch. Made from wheat endosperm, white flour is so refined that it is practically digested before you eat it, and it is converted into sugar as soon as it is consumed.

The refining process strips the grain of both water-soluble and water-insoluble fibers found in its bran and germ. These two nutritious segments of the grain also contain vitamins, proteins, and healthful oils. In whole grains, the presence of fiber slows down digestion and allows time for these important nutrients to be absorbed. Through refinement, many of these nutrients are lost. Digestion and absorption occur quickly, just as happens when you ingest simple carbohydrates.

Whole Grains

Whole-grain food products undergo less refinement and still contain healthful fiber. They take longer to digest and allow the body to fully absorb nutrients. Whole-wheat flour, brown rice, whole-grain pasta, and whole-grain cereals are just some of the foods available in most supermarkets. Because these foods convert more slowly to sugar and take longer to be absorbed, they are a healthier choice than refined, processed grains for your family.

Recipes

Pad Thai

*This simple and quick dish uses the flavors and textures of
Southeast Asia in a recipe perfect for a late-night dinner.*

INGREDIENTS | SERVES 4

¼ pound dried rice noodles

3 tablespoons rice vinegar

1 tablespoon fish sauce

2 tablespoons sugar

1 teaspoon Chinese chili paste with
  garlic

1 tablespoon peanut oil

3 cloves garlic, minced

1 egg, beaten

½ pound medium shrimp, peeled

2 cups mung bean sprouts

½ cup sliced green onions

¼ cup chopped peanuts

Bean Sprouts

It's easy to grow your own bean sprouts;
you'll find many books and lots of information online about the subject. You can also
find them in the grocery store, either fresh
in the produce aisle or canned. They are
very perishable. If you buy them fresh, use
them within two days or they may start to
spoil.

1. Place noodles in a large bowl and cover with warm
   water. Let soak until noodles are soft, about 20
   minutes. Drain noodles well and set aside.

2. In a small bowl, combine rice vinegar, fish sauce,
   sugar, and chili paste, and mix well; set aside. Have all
   ingredients ready.

3. In wok or large skillet, heat peanut oil over medium-
   high heat. Add garlic; cook until golden, about 15
   seconds. Add egg; stir-fry until set, about 30 seconds.
   Add shrimp and stir-fry until pink, about 2 minutes.

4. Add noodles to the wok, tossing with tongs until
   noodles soften and curl, about 1 minute. Add bean
   sprouts and green onions; stir-fry for 1 minute. Stir
   vinegar mixture and add to wok; stir-fry until mixture
   is hot, about 1–2 minutes longer. Sprinkle with peanuts
   and serve immediately.

PER SERVING Calories: 321.18 • Fat: 10.44 g • Protein: 15 g •
Sodium: 720.71 mg • Carbohydrates: 32 g • Fiber: 2 g

Amazing Amaranth Porridge with Amasake

Like millet and quinoa, amaranth is a gluten-free, protein-rich, alkaline grain. When cooked, amaranth becomes creamy porridge, which nourishes heart health.

INGREDIENTS | SERVES 2

½ cup amaranth
1½ cups water
Pinch sea salt
Amasake, to taste
½ medium umeboshi plum

1. Pour amaranth and water in saucepan and soak overnight. Add pinch of salt. Bring to boil, lower heat, and simmer, covered, 30 minutes.

2. Let sit off heat 5 minutes. Add amasake to taste.

3. Garnish with umeboshi plum.

PER SERVING Calories: 180 • Fat: 3 g • Protein: 7 g • Sodium: 138 mg • Carbohydrate: 32 g • Fiber: 3 g

Millet Corn Bread

This corn bread is a heart-healthy snack or harvest meal side dish. You can vary it by substituting quinoa for millet. Eat with brown rice syrup, apple butter, or almond butter.

INGREDIENTS | SERVES 20

2 cups cornmeal
1 cup spelt flour
¼ teaspoon salt
1½ cups cooked millet
½ cup safflower oil
1½ cups apple juice
½ cup almond milk

1. Preheat oven to 350°F. Mix dry ingredients together. Mix wet ingredients together in a separate bowl. Pour wet ingredients into dry and mix.

2. Pour mixture into 9" × 13" baking pan. Bake for 50 minutes. Slice and serve.

PER SERVING Calories: 180 • Fat: 8 g • Protein: 3 g • Sodium: 32 mg • Carbohydrate: 24 g • Fiber: 2 g

Quinoa Breakfast Congee

Congee is a porridge traditionally made with rice, and is primarily eaten as a breakfast food. It can even be enjoyed by individuals who are unable to chew due to illness or poor digestion. Congee takes a long time to cook, so it can be made in a rice cooker or slow cooker and cooked overnight.

INGREDIENTS | SERVES 4

¼ cup hijiki sea vegetable

½ onion

½ cup quinoa

½ cup brown rice

½ teaspoon sea salt

5 cups water

¼ cup toasted pumpkin seeds

Quinoa Tips

The versatility of quinoa is evident in its ability to be combined with beans, nuts, seeds, or vegetables. It also goes well with dried fruits or added to your favorite vegetable soups. Quinoa flour can be used to make cookies and muffins, and quinoa pasta tastes great with your favorite Italian sauce.

1. Soak hijiki in hot water for 10 minutes. Drain and set aside.

2. Chop onion and set aside.

3. Before going to bed, plug in a 1.5-quart slow cooker and add quinoa, rice, hijiki, onion, sea salt, and water. Set the temperature on low and cook overnight. (You can also use a rice cooker if it has a setting for "congee," as some do.)

4. In the morning, toast the pumpkin seeds in a dry skillet and set aside.

5. Stir the congee; spoon into individual serving bowls. Top with the pumpkin seeds and serve with cooked greens such as kale, spinach, or broccoli.

PER SERVING Calories: 193 • Fat: 2.5 g • Protein: 5 g • Sodium: 195 mg • Carbohydrates: 37 g • Fiber: 3 g

Quinoa Parsley Tabouleh

Make sure to seed the tomatoes for easier digestion,
but also to prevent excess liquid from making your tabouleh soggy.

INGREDIENTS | SERVES 6

1 cup quinoa
2 cups water or vegetable broth
½ teaspoon sea salt
1 cup fresh parsley
3 green onions
1 cup plum tomatoes
1 clove garlic
¼ cup extra-virgin olive oil
Juice of 1 fresh lemon
Sea salt, to taste

High-Protein Meal

Using quinoa in this traditional Middle Eastern dish is especially beneficial for individuals who cannot tolerate eating wheat couscous. This dish is high in protein; pair it with vegetables and a bean dish to round out its protein content. It is also light enough to serve as a side salad to a fish or chicken entrée.

1. In a heavy saucepan, combine quinoa, water (or vegetable broth), and sea salt; bring to a boil.

2. Reduce heat and simmer until all water is absorbed, about 15–20 minutes.

3. When quinoa is done, spoon into a large bowl and allow to cool.

4. While the grain is cooling, mince parsley and green onion; set aside.

5. Halve tomatoes lengthwise; scoop out seeds into a measuring cup or small bowl.

6. Chop tomatoes into small pieces; add to parsley and green onions.

7. Press and mince garlic; whisk it together in a small bowl with oil, lemon juice, and sea salt.

8. Strain and discard tomato seeds; add tomato liquid to lemon dressing.

9. Add parsley, green onion, and tomatoes to quinoa; toss well.

10. Add lemon dressing; mix well to combine all ingredients. Adjust seasonings with salt if needed.

PER SERVING Calories: 210 • Fat: 11 g • Carbohydrates: 23 g • Protein: 4 g • Sodium: 197 mg • Fiber: 2 g

Quinoa Black Bean Salad

The longer grain salads marinate, the better the flavors are absorbed by the ingredients. Make this salad the night before and take some to work for lunch the next day. Bring this salad to a potluck meal, and watch your friends enjoy something new and delicious.

INGREDIENTS | SERVES 8

1 cup quinoa

2 cups water

½ teaspoon sea salt

1 carrot

2 green onions

⅓ cup pumpkin seeds

½ cup parsley leaves

1 (14-ounce) can black beans

Juice of 1 lemon

1 clove garlic, minced

2 tablespoons apple cider vinegar

3 tablespoons extra-virgin olive oil

½ teaspoon salt

1. In a medium saucepan, combine quinoa, water, and ½ teaspoon sea salt. Cover, bring to a boil, reduce heat to low, and simmer until all water is absorbed, about 20 minutes.

2. When done, spoon into a large bowl and allow to cool.

3. Meanwhile, grate carrots, slice onions, toast pumpkin seeds, mince parsley, and rinse canned beans.

4. When quinoa is cool, add carrots, green onions, pumpkin seeds, black beans, and parsley; mix well.

5. In a small bowl, whisk together lemon, garlic, vinegar, oil, and salt.

6. Add vinaigrette; mix completely and allow to marinate a few minutes before serving.

PER SERVING Calories 190 • Fat 7 g • Protein 6 g • Sodium: 293 mg • Carbohydrates 26 g • Fiber 5 g

Toasting Pumpkin Seeds

Raw pumpkin seeds can be toasted in a dry skillet over medium-low heat. Keep them moving around by shaking the pan from time to time or stirring them with a wooden spoon. You'll know they are done when they've stopped popping or turned a golden brown.

Cilantro Chicken Tacos

By making your own taco shells at home, you significantly decrease the amount of fat in your taco meal.

INGREDIENTS | SERVES 6

2 cups corn or canola oil

6 (6") flour or whole-wheat tortillas

1 tablespoon olive oil

1 onion, chopped

3 boneless, skinless chicken breasts

1 green bell pepper, chopped

1 jalapeño pepper, minced

1 cup fresh salsa

⅓ cup chopped fresh cilantro

½ cup sour cream

1 cup chopped plum tomatoes

1 cup shredded lettuce

1 cup shredded jalapeño Monterey jack cheese

Cilantro and Coriander: Cousins

Two of the most widely used and loved herbs and spices in the world are derived from the same plant, *Coriandrum sativum*. The leaves of this plant are frequently referred to as cilantro, whereas the seeds are most commonly called coriander. Depending on the cuisine, the entire plant is used for its various flavors and aromas.

1. Pour corn or canola oil into a large deep saucepan and place over medium-high heat. Heat until oil temperature reaches 375°F. One at a time, fold tortillas in half and slip into the oil. Hold the taco shape with tongs as the tortilla fries, turning once during frying. Fry for 2–4 minutes on each side until the tortilla browns and puffs. Carefully remove from the oil, draining excess oil over the pot, and place tortilla on paper towels to drain. Repeat with remaining tortillas.

2. In large skillet, heat olive oil over medium heat. Add onion; cook and stir for 3 minutes. Meanwhile, cut chicken into 1" pieces. Add to skillet; cook and stir for 4 minutes longer. Add bell pepper and jalapeño; cook and stir for 1 minute longer.

3. Stir salsa and cilantro into chicken mixture; remove from heat. Make tacos with the cooled shells, chicken mixture, sour cream, plum tomatoes, lettuce, and shredded cheese.

PER SERVING Calories: 394 • Fat: 24 g • Protein: 21 g • Sodium: 532 mg • Carbohydrates: 25g • Fiber: 2.3 g

Sweet Red Salad with Strawberries and Beets

Colorful and nutritious, this vibrant red salad can be made with roasted or canned beets, or even raw grated beets, if you prefer.

INGREDIENTS | SERVES 4

3–4 small beets, chopped

Spinach or other green lettuce

1 cup sliced strawberries

½ cup chopped pecans

¼ cup olive oil

2 tablespoons red wine vinegar

2 tablespoons agave nectar

2 tablespoons orange juice

Salt and pepper, to taste

1. Boil beets until soft, about 20 minutes. Allow to cool completely.

2. In a large bowl, combine spinach, strawberries, pecans, and cooled beets.

3. In a separate small bowl, whisk together the olive oil, vinegar, agave nectar, and orange juice, and pour over salad, tossing well to coat.

4. Season generously with salt and pepper, to taste.

PER SERVING Calories: 295 • Fat: 24 g • Protein: 3 g • Sodium: 73 mg • Carbohydrates: 57 g • Fiber: 5 g

Sweet Potato Pie Pancakes

Enjoy this dish in early November to get excited about Thanksgiving dinner or a fall harvest celebration.

INGREDIENTS | SERVES 6

½ cup whole-wheat flour

¼ cup quick-cooking oatmeal

1 tablespoon Splenda

½ teaspoon baking powder

⅓ teaspoon baking soda

1½ cups canned sweet potatoes

2 tablespoons pecans, chopped

½ teaspoon cinnamon

1 teaspoon Splenda brown sugar

⅛ cup egg white substitute

1 cup skim milk

½ teaspoon vanilla extract

1. In a bowl, mix all dry ingredients together. In a separate bowl, mix all wet ingredients together. Gently fold dry ingredients into wet ingredients.

2. Coat skillet or griddle with nonstick spray. Pour ⅓ cup batter per pancake onto skillet.

3. Cook on medium-high heat until pancake develops bubbles on top. Flip the pancake and brown on the other side.

PER SERVING Calories: 122 • Fat: 1 g • Protein: 4 g • Sodium: 160 mg • Carbohydrates: 26 g • Fiber: 3 g

Baked Sweet Potato Fries

Tired of the same old sweet potatoes at Thanksgiving? Give these sweet, crispy fries a try!

INGREDIENTS | SERVES 6

2 pounds peeled sweet potatoes
2 teaspoons ground cinnamon
1 tablespoon olive oil

1. Preheat oven to 450°F. Cut potatoes into matchsticks, about ½" thick. Toss potatoes, cinnamon, and olive oil in a bowl.

2. Coat a large cookie sheet with nonstick spray. Bake for 25–30 minutes or until potatoes are fairly crispy.

PER SERVING Calories: 136 • Fat: 3 g • Protein: 2 g • Sodium: 14 mg • Carbohydrates: 27 g • Fiber: 4 g

Marinated Tempeh

Protein-rich Marinated Tempeh is a delicious dish for a vegan holiday feast. Or use tempeh in sandwiches, tacos, burritos, sushi, sautés, gravies, and salads. You can even add cooked vegetables and grains for delectable veggie tempeh burgers.

INGREDIENTS | SERVES 2

1 cup apple juice
¼ cup shoyu
1 slice ginger, chopped
2 cloves garlic
1 tablespoon brown rice vinegar
½ teaspoon cumin or ½ teaspoon mild curry
8 ounces tempeh
2 tablespoons sesame oil
1 batch Balsamic Vinegar Reduction (below)

1. Combine apple juice, shoyu, ginger, garlic, brown rice vinegar, and cumin or curry in a bowl.

2. Cut tempeh into ¼" thick strips. Soak tempeh overnight in marinade. In a skillet, pan fry tempeh in oil until golden brown on all sides. Add marinade to tempeh and cover skillet. Bring to boil, lower heat, and simmer for 15–20 minutes.

3. Remove tempeh from marinade and serve with Balsamic Vinegar Reduction.

PER SERVING Calories: 511 • Fat: 19g • Protein: 22g • Sodium: 295mg • Carbohydrate: 56g • Fiber: 0g

Balsamic Vinegar Reduction

Bring 2 cups of good quality balsamic vinegar to boil. Reduce heat and simmer, uncovered, until sauce is reduced to ⅔ cup. Stir often to prevent sticking. The vinegar naturally becomes sweeter when reduced.

Indian Curried Lentil Soup

Similar to a traditional Indian lentil dal recipe, but with added vegetables to make it into an entrée, this lentil soup is perfect as is, or pair it with rice or some warmed Indian flatbread.

INGREDIENTS | SERVES 4

1 onion, diced

1 carrot, sliced

3 whole cloves

2 tablespoons vegan margarine

1 teaspoon cumin

1 teaspoon turmeric

1 cup yellow or green lentils

2¾ cup vegetable broth

2 large tomatoes, chopped

1 teaspoon salt

¼ teaspoon black pepper

1 teaspoon lemon juice

1. In a large soup or stock pot, sauté the onion, carrot, and cloves in margarine until onions are just turning soft, about 3 minutes. Add cumin and turmeric and toast for 1 minute, stirring constantly to avoid burning.

2. Reduce heat to medium low and add lentils, vegetable broth, tomatoes, and salt. Bring to a simmer, cover, and cook for 35–40 minutes, or until lentils are done.

3. Season with black pepper and lemon juice just before serving.

PER SERVING Calories: 265 • Fat: 6 g • Protein: 14 g • Sodium: 1,328 mg • Carbohydrates: 30 g • Fiber: 17 g

Vegan Tempeh "Meatballs"

This vegan version of meatballs makes a great appetizer or burgers. Lentil purée and brown rice help hold "meatballs" together. Tempeh balls can be baked or rolled in cornmeal and pan fried.

INGREDIENTS | SERVES 6

¼ cup onion, minced

1 clove garlic, crushed

¼ cup carrot, grated

¼ cup celery, minced

¼ teaspoon coriander

1 batch Marinated Tempeh (see following)

½ cup cooked brown lentils

1½ cups cooked brown rice

¼ cup safflower oil

1. In a skillet, sauté onion, garlic, carrot, celery, and coriander until cooked.

2. Crumble tempeh and add to the skillet with brown lentils and brown rice.

3. Form into balls. In a skillet, pan fry balls in oil until browned, about 10 minutes.

PER SERVING Calories: 280 • Fat: 18 g • Protein: 10 g • Sodium: 133 mg • Carbohydrate: 21 g • Fiber: 3 g

Luscious Lima Beans and Corn

Succotash is a Southern dish traditionally made with lima beans and dried corn that is often served at Thanksgiving. Green beans or kidney beans can be used in place of lima beans. Vegetables such as sun-dried tomatoes, squash, edamame, onions, red bell peppers, and peas can be included.

INGREDIENTS | SERVES 6

1 cup lima beans, soaked
Spring water, as needed
1 stamp-sized piece kombu, soaked
3 cups fresh corn kernels
1 teaspoon olive oil
2 teaspoons sweet white miso
¼ cup chives, chopped

1. Drain beans. Place beans in a saucepan and cover with water. Bring to boil and remove foam. Add kombu, lower heat, and simmer for 1½ hours or until tender, adding more water if needed.

2. Add corn, olive oil, and sweet white miso. Simmer for 5 minutes.

3. Garnish with chives.

PER SERVING Calories: 184 • Fat: 3 g • Protein: 9 g • Sodium: 68 mg • Carbohydrate: 34 g • Fiber: 8 g

Easy Miso Noodle Soup

This delicious soup relaxes and nourishes the body after a long day. White-colored miso will give a lighter taste than dark red or brown miso. The darker the miso, the longer it has been fermented and the more live enzymes it will provide. Feel free to add other vegetables or a small filet of fish to the soup.

INGREDIENTS | SERVES 4

½ onion
2 medium carrots
2 green onions
4–6 cups vegetable broth or water
1 tablespoon dried wakame
1 cube firm tofu
4 teaspoons mellow white miso
1 (8-ounce) package cooked soba noodles
4 tablespoons pumpkin seeds, toasted

1. Cut the onion in thin half-moon slices; julienne carrots into matchstick shapes; slice green onions diagonally.

2. Heat broth; and add onion, carrot, wakame, and tofu. Simmer until onion is just tender.

3. Ladle broth into individual bowls; dissolve 1 teaspoon of miso into each.

4. Add ½ cup noodles to each bowl; ladle in soup with vegetables and tofu.

5. Serve topped with pumpkin seeds and sliced green onions.

PER SERVING Calories: 180 • Fat: 3.5 g • Carbohydrates: 30 g • Protein: 10 g • Sodium: 253 mg • Fiber: 5 g

Spinach and Ricotta Mini-Quiches

*Top these mini-quiches with a slice of tomato and sprinkle on some shredded cheese
to add a nice touch of color and great flavor.*

INGREDIENTS | SERVES 5

10 ounces chopped frozen spinach

2 eggs

1 cup skim ricotta cheese

1 cup low-fat shredded mozzarella
cheese

1. Preheat oven to 350°F. Place cupcake liners in 12-hole cupcake tin.

2. Heat spinach in microwave according to package directions, until soft and warm.

3. Whip the eggs and add the spinach. Blend together.

4. Fold in the ricotta and shredded mozzarella cheese.

5. Fill each cup with egg-spinach mixture, about ½" per cup.

6. Bake 30–35 minutes.

PER SERVING Calories: 175 • Fat: 10 g • Protein: 16 g • Sodium: 273 mg • Carbohydrates: 5 g • Fiber: 1.8 g

CHAPTER 5

Focus on Fiber

Americans tend to skimp when it comes to "whole" fiber intake. Many products on the supermarket shelves contain "isolated fiber" (the fiber food manufactures add to foods that would not naturally contain fiber), which does not provide the same benefits. Sources of fiber that support weight loss, satiety, heart health, and digestion derive from natural plant sources: vegetables, fruit, and whole grains. A healthy diet contains 25–38 grams per day of fiber, from a variety of sources. Fiber's ability to control blood sugars and hunger makes it an important part of a meal or snack.

Soluble and Insoluble Fiber

As was discussed earlier, there are two kinds of fiber: water-soluble and water-insoluble. Both are necessary for good health. Water-soluble fibers have been shown to help lower blood cholesterol levels when included in a low-fat diet. Low-density lipoprotein (LDL) cholesterol levels appear to drop more when water-soluble fiber is part of your diet than when you eat a low-fat diet alone. In addition, water-soluble fibers slow the rate of digestion, which in turn increases the rate of nutrient absorption. The longer a food remains in the intestines, the more nutrients can be absorbed from it. Oats have the most soluble fiber of any grain, followed by barley and brown rice. Soluble fiber can also be found in legumes, citrus fruit, berries, and apples.

Insoluble fiber, such as cellulose, comes from the skin, stems, and seeds of plants. It is linked to lower risk and slower progression of cardiovascular disease. Because it keeps waste moving through the intestines, insoluble fiber may help prevent colon cancer by reducing the time cancer-causing agents are in the intestine. Fiber swells as it absorbs water, which delays the emptying of the stomach so you eat less. Not only is this good for absorption, it makes you feel full longer. The extra chewing it takes to break down fiber forces you to eat more slowly, too, which gives your stomach time to tell your brain it's full.

Bran and whole-grain foods that still include the grain's outer hull, such as brown rice, are good sources of insoluble fiber. Nuts, fruit in its skin, and vegetables, including cabbage, celery, carrots, beets, and cauliflower, are also excellent sources of insoluble fiber.

Daily Requirements

The average adult needs about three cups of vegetables and four to five cups of grains every day. Most Americans get nowhere near that amount. As a general rule, one-third of your plate at every meal should be filled with fiber-rich grains, and every snack should include either fiber-filled fruit, vegetables, or grains.

As a country, we eat only 10 percent of the amount of fiber we ate at the turn of the twentieth century. Americans eat a lot of wheat, but it is made into highly refined flour and mixed with refined sugars and hydrogenated oils until your body no longer recognizes it as grain. Refined grains are partially responsible for the epidemic of weight gain, Type 2 diabetes, and cardiovascular disease. In addition, lack of fiber in the modern diet seems to be linked to gastrointestinal disorders, including several forms of cancer.

Increased intake of fiber can reduce these risks dramatically. As an added bonus, fiber sources also contain vitamins, minerals, protein, and limited oils.

Fiber Supplements

Fiber supplements are often prescribed for constipation and other bowel disorders. But these prescriptions are generally meant to be used for a limited time, until the conditions are alleviated. Lack of exercise, insufficient fluid intake, and a lack of fiber intake all contribute to bowel malfunctions, as do some medications and surgical procedures.

It's easy to get too much fiber from supplements. This is problematic, as fiber binds to some minerals, including calcium and iron, preventing absorption. The conclusion is that fiber is best taken naturally. It's not hard to get the fiber you need. Choose bread that has at least two grams of fiber per slice. Eat high-fiber snacks such as popcorn and fresh veggies. For breakfast, add berries and dried fruit to high-fiber cereal. By getting your fiber this way, you also get all the other nutrients associated with those foods, which you need every day anyway.

Natural Sources of Fiber

The following list includes some common grains that you can use to make pilafs similar to those in this chapter's recipes. They are not difficult to cook, and they offer much more in the way of flavor than plain, refined white rice. The basic method of cooking grain is to boil it in water. The ratio of water to grain varies, but it is generally two-and-a-half to three parts water to one part grain. Boil the water, then add the grain, and simmer over low heat with the lid on to trap the steam. This tenderizes the grain by encouraging absorption of water. You can also cook grain as you would pasta, in a large pot of boiling water, straining out the grain when tender. This method loses some nutrients, but it is convenient if the optimal water-to-grain ratio is unknown.

Simply boiling grains cooks them, but their flavor is greatly enhanced by toasting. Several recipes in this chapter use a small amount of oil to toast the grain until it's brown and fragrant, giving it a nutty, rich flavor.

- **Amaranth:** This tiny grain, grown at high altitude, originated in the Andes and Himalayas. It is commonly popped like popcorn, and bound together with honey, like an ancient Rice Krispies treat.
- **Barley:** This grain is less popular than it used to be. People rarely eat it except in soup, but it can make delicious side dishes and casseroles. Pearled or polished barley has the bran removed. Hulled barley has the bran intact and is the more healthful choice.
- **Buckwheat:** This is not really a grain, but the seed of an herb native to Russia. It is commonly ground into flour and used in a variety of breads. It is also known as kasha, a toasted buckwheat groat that is cooked like rice.
- **Bulgur:** These wheat kernels have been steamed, dried, and crushed. They do not require cooking but need only be soaked in cold water. Bulgur is the base of Middle Eastern tabouleh salad.
- **Couscous:** This is not a grain, but a coarse granular semolina, which is a flour made from protein-rich wheat called durum. Couscous cooks quickly, and is a terrific vehicle for flavorful sauces and stews. It is usually associated with the cuisine of Morocco.
- **Cracked wheat:** This wheat is crushed with the bran intact. It is not pre-steamed like bulgur, so it must be cooked in boiling water like rice.
- **Kamut:** This is an ancient strain of wheat, whose kernels are more than twice the size of modern wheat kernels and contain a greater amount of protein. It can be made into pilafs, kneaded into breads, or ground into flour.
- **Millet:** Used mostly as bird seed in the United States, this small grain is a staple food in much of the world, due to its high protein content and pleasantly mild flavor. It cooks up soft and delicate.
- **Oats:** Most Americans eat oatmeal from rolled, quick-cooking oats. But oats are also available steel cut, as groats (grains that are hulled and crushed), which provide more nourishment, or as flour.
- **Quinoa:** This tiny grain has gained recent popularity, but it is actually an ancient food the Incas and Aztecs consumed. It is extremely high in protein and easy to cook, and it has a pleasant crunch.

- **Rye:** Closely related to barley and wheat, rye is available rolled like oats or as rye berries, in which the grain is whole with the bran removed. Rye flour is commonly used in bread making, although it contains no gluten.
- **Spelt:** This is an ancient relative of wheat, native to southern Europe. Spelt has more protein than common wheat and, like kamut, has huge nutty grains.
- **Teff:** A tiny grain from Africa, teff is high in protein, calcium, and iron. It is eaten as porridge or ground into flour, and it is used to make the Ethiopian bread injera.
- **Triticale:** This is a nutritious hybrid of wheat and rye, available in whole-grain flour.
- **Wheat berries:** These are whole grains of wheat stripped of their outer hulls.

Fruit and Vegetable Fiber

The more skins and seeds you eat with your fruits and veggies, the more fiber you'll get. Fruits and veggies that are mostly skin and seeds—raspberries, blackberries, corn, kiwi, cucumbers, figs, and dried fruits—provide lots of fiber. Stems are good too, and although you may not relish the thought of eating a stem, consider that celery and asparagus are nothing but stem.

All green leafy vegetables are loaded with fiber—you can see it in the veins of their leaves. Artichokes, brussels sprouts, green beans, and onions are all good sources, too. And the sweet potato is a fiber gold mine.

Keep plenty of these fiber-rich fruits and vegetables on hand. Wash and cut them into serving sizes to encourage healthy snacking. Make fresh salads part of everyday eating, and use fresh and dried fruits to combat a sweet tooth.

Recipes

Spanish Artichoke and Zucchini Paella

Traditional Spanish paellas are always cooked with saffron, but this version with zucchini, artichokes, and bell peppers uses turmeric instead to produce the same golden hue at a fraction of the cost of saffron.

INGREDIENTS | SERVES 4

3 cloves garlic, minced

1 yellow onion, diced

2 tablespoons olive oil

1 cup white rice

1 (15-ounce) can diced or crushed tomatoes

1 green bell pepper, chopped

1 red or yellow bell pepper, chopped

½ cup artichoke hearts, chopped

2 zucchini, sliced

2 cups vegetable broth

1 tablespoon paprika

½ teaspoon turmeric

¾ teaspoon parsley

½ teaspoon salt

1. In a largest skillet you can find, heat garlic and onions in olive oil for 3–4 minutes, until onions are almost soft. Add rice, stirring well to coat, and heat for another minute, stirring to prevent burning.

2. Add tomatoes, bell peppers, artichokes, and zucchini, stirring to combine. Add vegetable broth and remaining ingredients, cover, and simmer for 15–20 minutes, or until rice is done.

PER SERVING Calories: 260 • Fat: 1 g • Protein: 7 g • Sodium: 1,016 mg • Carbohydrates: 44 g • Fiber: 6 g

Zucchini Casserole

This casserole isn't just a delicious side dish, it is filling enough to serve as an entire vegetarian entrée. As an entrée it should provide three servings.

INGREDIENTS | SERVES 6

1 clove fresh garlic, minced

1 teaspoon olive oil

4 large zucchini, sliced

1 cup white mushrooms, sliced

1 (15-ounce) can Italian-style stewed tomatoes

½ cup Italian-style bread crumbs

¼ cup shredded low-fat Parmesan cheese

¼ cup shredded low-fat mozzarella cheese

1. Coat a 9" × 13" baking dish with nonstick spray.

2. Place garlic and olive oil in a large skillet and sauté for 6 minutes on medium heat.

3. Add zucchini to skillet and sauté for 5 minutes. Add mushrooms and sauté for 5 minutes. Remove from burner, add tomatoes, and stir.

4. Pour veggies into the baking dish. Cover veggies with bread crumbs. Sprinkle cheeses over bread crumbs.

5. Bake at 350°F for 15 minutes or until cheese melts.

PER SERVING Calories: 111 • Fat: 2 g • Protein: 7 g • Sodium: 486 mg • Carbohydrates: 17 g • Fiber: 3 g

Coriander Carrots

Rich with beta-carotene, carrots make a wonderful side dish,
and these are especially fragrant and flavorful.

INGREDIENTS | SERVES 6

1 tablespoon olive oil

1 onion, chopped

1 cup water

1 bay leaf

½ teaspoon salt

1½ pounds carrots, thickly sliced

¼ cup dried currants

1 tablespoon butter

2 teaspoons ground coriander

2 tablespoons lemon juice

3 tablespoons minced flat-leaf parsley

1. Heat oil in a large saucepan over medium heat. Add onion; cook and stir until crisp-tender, about 4 minutes. Add water, bay leaf, salt, carrots, and currants, and bring to a simmer.

2. Cover pan, reduce heat to low, and simmer for 10–15 minutes or until carrots are tender when tested with a fork.

3. Drain carrots, remove bay leaf, and return saucepan to heat. Add butter, coriander, lemon juice, and parsley; cook and stir over low heat for 2–3 minutes or until carrots are glazed. Serve immediately.

PER SERVING Calories: 95 • Fat: 3 g • Protein: 1.6 g • Sodium: 254 mg • Carbohydrates: 16 g • Fiber: 4 g

Serve 'Em Up Right

Coriander and bay leaf add a nice spicy touch to tender carrots. Serve this carrot dish with grilled chicken or rice dishes, or as a side for your Thanksgiving meal.

Garden Quesadillas

Quesadillas are made from two tortillas with a filling, toasted on a griddle until crisp.

INGREDIENTS | SERVES 4–6

2 tablespoons olive oil
1 onion, chopped
1 red bell pepper, chopped
½ cup chopped mushrooms
1 cup fresh salsa
8 whole-wheat tortillas
1 cup baby spinach leaves
1 cup shredded pepper jack cheese

1. In a medium skillet, heat 1 tablespoon olive oil over medium heat. Add onion; cook and stir until crisp-tender, about 4 minutes. Add bell pepper and mushrooms; cook and stir for 2–4 minutes longer until tender. Drain and combine in medium bowl with salsa.

2. Arrange tortillas on work surface. Top half of the tortillas with some of the baby spinach leaves and spoon onion mixture on top. Top with cheese, then with remaining tortillas, and press down gently.

3. Heat griddle or skillet over medium heat. Brush with remaining olive oil, then grill quesadillas, turning once and pressing down occasionally with spatula, until cheese melts and tortillas are toasted. Cut into quarters and serve immediately.

PER SERVING Calories: 297 • Fat: 16 g • Protein: 11 g • Sodium: 562 mg • Carbohydrates: 29 g • Fiber: 3.7 g

Summer Asparagus

Asparagus combined with other fresh vegetables makes a wonderful and easy side dish that pairs beautifully with any main dish.

1 pound asparagus spears

2 tablespoons butter

¼ cup chopped green onion

½ cup chopped tomato

1 avocado, peeled and chopped

Ain't Asparagus Great?

Asparagus is low in calories, contains no cholesterol, and is very low in sodium. It is also a good source of folic acid, potassium, and dietary fiber. Need another reason to eat it? It tastes delicious!

1. Wash asparagus spears and snap off tough ends. Place in boiling salted water; cook for 3–4 minutes or until just crisp-tender. Drain in a colander and arrange on serving plate.

2. Meanwhile, in a small saucepan combine butter with green onion; cook and stir over medium heat until crisp-tender, about 3 minutes. Remove from heat and stir in tomato and avocado. Pour over asparagus and serve.

PER SERVING Calories: 152 • Fat: 13 g • Protein: 3.4 g • Sodium: 66 mg • Carbohydrates: 9 g • Fiber: 5.4 g

Citrus Green Beans

Tender and crisp green beans are perked up with lemon and orange juice in this simple side dish.

1½ pounds fresh green beans

3 tablespoons butter

3 cloves garlic, minced

2 tablespoons lemon juice

¼ cup orange juice

1 teaspoon grated orange zest

1 teaspoon salt

⅛ teaspoon white pepper

1. Bring a large pot of salted water to a boil. Trim green beans and rinse. Add to water and bring back to a simmer. Cook for 3 minutes, then drain.

2. In a large skillet, melt butter and add garlic. Cook over medium heat until garlic is fragrant, about 2 minutes. Add green beans; cook and stir for 3–5 minutes or until beans are crisp-tender. Stir in lemon juice, orange juice, orange zest, salt, and pepper, and heat through.

PER SERVING Calories: 94 • Fat: 6 g • Protein: 1 g • Sodium: 449 mg • Carbohydrates: 10 g • Fiber: 1.2 g

Scallion Tabouleh

Bulgur, or cracked wheat, is a nutritious and tasty side dish that's chewy and nutty. It is high in fiber, which fills you up and keeps you satisfied for hours.

INGREDIENTS | SERVES 8

1 cup bulgur

2 cups boiling water

½ cup chopped flat-leaf parsley

⅓ cup raisins

⅓ cup dried currants

½ cup chopped green onion

¼ cup lime juice

1 tablespoon olive oil

½ teaspoon salt

⅛ teaspoon pepper

Currants

Currants are small berry-like fruits most commonly found in red and black varieties. The tart flavor of the red currant is slightly stronger than the black. Because of their strong flavor, currants are usually cooked, dried, or made into jellies, rather than being eaten fresh.

1. In a medium bowl, combine bulgur and boiling water. Cover and let stand for 20 minutes, or according to package directions, until tender.

2. Drain to remove excess moisture, if necessary, then transfer to a serving bowl. Add parsley, raisins, currants, and green onion; toss to mix well. In a small bowl, stir together lime juice, oil, salt, and pepper. Add to the bulgur mixture, toss well, and serve.

3. Mixture can be heated in the microwave, if desired. Microwave on 50 percent power for 2–3 minutes, remove, and stir. Continue microwaving on 50 percent power for 1-minute intervals until mixture is steaming. Let stand for 5 minutes, then serve.

PER SERVING Calories: 130 • Fat: 2 g • Protein: 1.3 g • Sodium: 162 mg • Carbohydrates: 14 g • Fiber: 2 g

Fall Minestrone Soup

Minestrone is the Italian name for a thick and hearty soup that often consists of legumes, veggies, rice, and/or pasta. The ingredients in this soup change with the season. Whichever vegetable is growing at the time gets used!

INGREDIENTS | SERVES 6

½ cup yellow onions, chopped
1 clove fresh garlic, minced
½ teaspoon all-purpose seasoning
1 cup frozen peas
1 cup squash, sliced
1 cup green beans
1 cup carrots, sliced
2 cups white beans, cooked
1 cup chickpeas, cooked
1 cup frozen spinach
½ cup whole-wheat pasta
1 teaspoon oregano
¼ teaspoon black pepper
1 chicken bouillon cube
3 cups water

1. Combine all ingredients in a large saucepan. Cook on medium-high heat for 15 minutes.

2. Reduce heat to low, simmer for another 10 minutes, then serve.

PER SERVING Calories: 210 • Fat: 1 g • Protein: 13 g • Sodium: 209 mg • Carbohydrates: 39 g • Fiber: 9 g

Veggie-Stuffed Zucchini

Stuff the zucchini with any vegetables you like.
The vegetables in this recipe can easily be substituted with your favorites.

INGREDIENTS | SERVES 4

4 medium zucchini
1 teaspoon salt
2 teaspoons vegan margarine
2 teaspoons vegetable oil
1 onion, chopped
1 clove garlic, crushed
½ cup chickpeas
2 tablespoons flour
1 teaspoon ground coriander
1 potato, peeled, cooked, and diced
1 cup green peas
2 tablespoons chopped cilantro

1. Preheat oven to 375°F.

2. Cut each zucchini in half lengthwise and scoop out the pulp. Place each half with the open side up on a shallow roasting pan and sprinkle with salt.

3. Heat margarine and oil in a skillet over medium heat. Add onion and garlic; sauté for 4 minutes, then stir in chickpeas, flour, coriander, potato, peas, and cilantro.

4. Spoon ¼ of potato mixture into each zucchini half and cover with foil.

5. Bake for 15 minutes or until zucchini is tender.

PER SERVING Calories: 205 • Fat: 5 g • Protein: 8 g • Sodium: 68 mg • Carbohydrates: 35 g • Fiber: 5 g

Edamame Salad

If you can't find shelled edamame, try this recipe with lima beans instead.

INGREDIENTS | SERVES 4

2 cups frozen shelled edamame, thawed and drained

1 red or yellow bell pepper, diced

¾ cup corn kernels

3 tablespoons chopped fresh cilantro (optional)

3 tablespoons olive oil

2 tablespoons red wine vinegar

1 teaspoon soy sauce

1 teaspoon chili powder

2 teaspoons lemon or lime juice

Salt and pepper, to taste

1. Combine edamame, bell pepper, corn, and cilantro in a large bowl.

2. Whisk together the olive oil, vinegar, soy sauce, chili powder, and lemon or lime juice, and combine with the edamame. Add salt and pepper to taste.

3. Chill for at least 1 hour before serving.

PER SERVING Calories: 246 • Fat: 16 g • Protein: 10 g • Sodium: 133 mg • Carbohydrates: 42 g • Fiber: 9 g

Cucumber Cilantro Salad

Cool cucumbers and creamy yogurt are coupled with a dash of cayenne pepper for a salad that keeps you guessing.

INGREDIENTS | SERVES 2–3

4 cucumbers, diced

2 tomatoes, chopped

½ red onion, diced small

1 cup soy yogurt, plain or lemon flavored

1 tablespoon lemon juice

2 tablespoons chopped fresh cilantro

Salt and pepper, to taste

¼ teaspoon cayenne (optional)

1. Toss together all ingredients, stirring well to combine.

2. Chill for at least 2 hours before serving, to allow flavors to marinate. Toss again just before serving.

PER SERVING Calories: 134 • Fat: 2 g • Protein: 6 g • Sodium: 23 mg • Carbohydrates: 36 g • Fiber: 4 g

Roasted Brussels Sprouts with Apples

Brussels sprouts are surprisingly delicious when prepared properly, so if you have bad memories of being force-fed soggy, limp baby cabbages as a child, don't let it stop you from trying this recipe.

INGREDIENTS | SERVES 4

2 cups Brussels sprouts, chopped into quarters

8 whole cloves garlic, peeled

2 tablespoons olive oil

2 tablespoons balsamic vinegar

¾ teaspoon salt

½ teaspoon black pepper

2 apples, chopped

1. Preheat oven to 425°F.

2. Arrange Brussels sprouts and garlic on a single layer on a baking sheet. Drizzle with olive oil and balsamic vinegar, and season with salt and pepper. Roast for 10–12 minutes, tossing once.

3. Remove tray from oven and add apples, tossing gently to combine. Roast for 10 more minutes, or until apples are soft, tossing once again.

PER SERVING Calories: 143 • Fat: 7 g • Protein: 2 g • Sodium: 451 mg • Carbohydrates: 19 g • Fiber: 4 g

Tuscan Bean Soup

Tuscan cuisine combines a mixture of vegetables with the flavor of Mediterranean aromatic herbs.

INGREDIENTS | SERVES 6

1 clove fresh garlic, minced

2 cups zucchini, sliced

1 teaspoon oregano

½ cup bell peppers, diced

2 cups tomatoes, diced

1 teaspoon all-purpose seasoning

1 teaspoon cumin

½ cup carrots, sliced

1 cup red wine

3 cups white beans, cooked

4 cups chicken broth

½ teaspoon black pepper

1 tablespoon tomato paste

½ cup celery, sliced

1. Combine all ingredients in a large saucepan. Cook on medium-high heat for 15 minutes.

2. Reduce heat to low, simmer for another 10 minutes, then serve.

PER SERVING Calories: 242 • Fat: 4 g • Protein: 14 g • Sodium: 595 mg • Carbohydrates: 33 g • Fiber: 9 g

Black Bean and Chicken Sausage Stew

Make this stew to serve your guests and family, take along to a potluck dinner, or freeze in individual containers for future use. Otherwise, halve the ingredients to serve six, and season with salt to taste.

INGREDIENTS | SERVES 12

½ pound dried black beans

7 cups water

3-inch piece kombu sea vegetable

1 onion

1 green pepper

2 carrots

1 medium sweet potato

3 cloves garlic

1 package organic chicken sausage (6 links)

¼ cup extra-virgin olive oil

2 teaspoons cumin powder

1 teaspoon sea salt

2 tablespoons kuzu-root powder

Methods of Cooking

You can speed up the process of cooking your beans by using a pressure cooker, which will cut the time in half. If you do not have the time to cook dried beans, use canned black beans and prepare the vegetables with a quick sauté, then add all the ingredients to a slow cooker and cook on high for 3 hours or on low for 5–6 hours.

1. In a large saucepan or pressure cooker, cover beans with water and soak overnight. In the morning, drain, return beans to pot, and add 7 cups water. Add kombu to beans; bring water to boil, reduce heat; and simmer until beans are tender, about 1 hour.

2. Meanwhile, chop onion, green pepper, and carrots; peel and chop sweet potato; mince garlic. Slice sausage links and chop into bite-size pieces.

3. In a large Dutch oven, heat oil; sauté onion, pepper, carrots, and garlic until almost tender. Add cumin powder to onion mixture; stir well to combine. Add chopped sausage; allow to cook another 3 minutes. Add cooked black beans and liquid to sausage mixture; stir well.

4. Stir in sea salt; bring mixture to a boil, reduce heat, cover, and simmer until vegetables are cooked and tender, about 20 minutes, stirring occasionally.

5. In a small glass or measuring cup, dissolve kuzu-root powder with a small amount of water. Slowly add to black bean stew, stirring as you do so. It should begin to thicken immediately, so watch for level of thickness desired.

6. Cover and allow to simmer another minute or two. Remove from heat; adjust seasonings; and serve.

PER SERVING Calories: 150 • Fat: 6 g • Protein: 5 g • Sodium: 269 mg • Carbohydrates: 18 g • Fiber: 3 g

Aduki Beans, Kombu, and Squash

This dish nourishes the middle organs and the kidneys, and aids diabetes and hypoglycemia. Experiment with various squashes, carrots, sautéed onion, and tempeh.

INGREDIENTS | SERVES 4

1 cup aduki beans, soaked in 4 cups water

1 stamp-sized piece kombu, soaked

1 cup kabocha squash, large chunks

Shoyu (soy sauce), to taste

½ cup mochi, grated, optional

¼ cup parsley, chopped

Preparing Beans for Cooking

Preparing beans before cooking makes them more digestible. First, remove stones from beans. Rinse beans under cool water, and soak 6–8 hours. Bring beans and water to boil, and remove foam. Then, cook beans with kombu to soften beans and balance oils.

1. In a heavy pot, add aduki beans and soaking water. Bring to boil and skim off foam. Add kombu and squash. Lower heat, and simmer, covered, 1½ hours. Add more water, if necessary, to cover beans.

2. Add shoyu and simmer another 15 minutes.

3. Stir grated mochi into hot beans to melt. Garnish with parsley.

PER SERVING Calories: 175 • Fat: 0 g • Protein: 10 g • Sodium: 27 mg • Carbohydrate: 34 g • Fiber: 7 g

CHAPTER 6

Sweet, Sweet Sugar

Refined sugar causes your body to crave more refined foods, suppresses your immune system, and causes your energy levels to spike then crash. There are more than twenty different names for sugar, most being refined, in our sweet but poor national diet. The average American consumes about 150 pounds of sugar annually. A person could lose fifteen pounds in one year just by cutting out sugary sodas. If you would like to take control of your food cravings and eliminate excess weight, get your sweet fix in other, more nutritionally beneficial ways. Begin by learning the difference between "added" and "natural" sugars.

How Your Body Uses Sugar

Your body is designed to utilize the sugar in food as energy. Carbohydrates found in natural sugars and starches are broken down into their simple molecular components so they may be absorbed and converted to energy. In addition, these foods have other nutrients that your body needs and uses: vitamins, minerals, proteins, fats, and fiber.

Unfortunately, refined sugar, or sucrose, has no nutritional value. Although it is derived from plants (sugar cane and beets), it has been depleted of all other nutrients. What remains is pure carbohydrate in a form the human body was not built to utilize.

All these empty calories (foods that contain calories, but offer no viable nutrition are said to contain "empty calories") cannot possibly be used, and therefore are stored in the liver as glycogen. When the liver is full, excess glycogen is taken to the blood in the form of fatty acids and transported for storage all over the body, but particularly to areas that are relatively inactive: your belly, butt, breasts, and thighs. When these areas are full, the fatty acids are distributed between your organs, reducing their ability to function.

FACT

Sugar cane originated in the Pacific Islands, then migrated to Asia, the Middle East, and India. The Crusaders brought "sweet salt" back from their expeditions, and by the 1400s sugar cane plantations were in full production throughout the Mediterranean. By the 1600s, production began in the Caribbean, where it flourished. In the 1700s, beets became a popular sugar source when a British blockade denied Napoleon his Caribbean imports.

Your body reacts so strongly to a sudden influx of pure carbohydrate that you can physically feel a rush of energy. Unlike the sugar you get from fruits, milk, or honey, refined sugar is metabolized instantly. Once your body uses up the sugar, it craves more and sends you into withdrawal. If you don't consume more, you experience the inevitable crash. Your body reacts to what is essentially poison by sending nutrients to help keep you in balance. Vitamins, minerals, and enzymes rush to the rescue, resulting in depletion of these nutrients throughout the body.

Sure, carbohydrates are essential for good nutrition. But you were never meant to eat them in a refined state. Your body needs the full benefit of the nutrients that come with a piece of fruit or even a taste of honey. These natural foods take time to digest, entering the body slowly, so they can be put to use where and when they are needed.

Curbing Your Sugar Intake

Human babies respond to sugar quite early. The taste is innately pleasant because the calorie-rich carbohydrates are an essential energy source for humans. The taste for all things sweet develops as you age, but society has helped it along. In the twentieth century the demand for sugar skyrocketed. Americans went from an annual consumption of a mere five pounds in the 1890s to the current intake of 150 pounds. How did this happen?

Soda pop is a major contributor to our increased sugar intake. Sugar-laden beverages won't quench your thirst. They are nothing more than liquid candy. But many Americans consume sodas with every meal, and between meals as well. Kids can even buy sodas at school.

Sugar absorbs water. In baking, this phenomenon helps keep products moist. In your body, it just makes you thirsty. As a result, drinking beverages with sugar to quench your thirst is counterproductive. This, coupled with the craving for sugar that comes after sugar is consumed, equals a guaranteed repeat customer for the soda pop companies.

ESSENTIAL

Cats, from large jungle cats down to domestic house cats, are unable to recognize sweetness. In the wild, they're strictly meat eaters, so they have evolved without the sweet taste receptor. You can test it by offering your pets a bowl of water and a bowl of sugar water. Dogs, however, will feed their sweet teeth.

The other contributor to America's skyrocketing sugar consumption is hidden sugar. Whether you realize it or not, sugar is in almost everything you eat. Sure, you know it's in the obvious stuff, such as soda and cookies and candy. But it's also in ketchup, mayonnaise, salad dressings, fruit juice, bread, cereal, soups, pizza, pasta, yogurt, and cheese. And when foods are marketed as fat-free, there's a good possibility sugar is increased to raise palatability.

Check the labels of the food in your cupboard. Unless a product is specifically labeled sugar-free, chances are it will have sugar in it. But be sure to look carefully. Sugar goes by other names, including dextrose, glucose, fructose, lactose, corn syrup, sorghum, galactose, invert sugar, and malt or maltose.

Refined Versus Natural Sugar

You cannot escape all the sugar in foods, nor should you. You need it for survival, and let's not forget that sugar is yummy. But some sugars are better for you than others. You can get the sugar you need, eliminate what you don't, and still have a pleasurable life.

Granulated Sugar

Commonly referred to as white sugar or table sugar, it is made both from sugar cane and sugar beets. They are generally interchangeable, although cane sugar is preferable for candy work, as it tends to crystallize less than beet sugar.

Brown Sugar

This is white sugar that has molasses added to it, although traditionally brown sugar was less refined than white table sugar. In today's manufacturing process, it is more economical to refine all sugar, then add molasses (which is removed during refinement) back in to make brown sugar. Light brown sugar has less molasses, and less flavor, than the dark brown variety. Otherwise, they are interchangeable and their use should be determined by your taste preferences.

Molasses

A by-product of the sugar refinement process, molasses is widely used for its flavor and color. Unsulfured molasses is considered the finest quality and is made by boiling ripened sugar cane. Sulfured molasses is made from green sugar cane that is treated during extraction with sulfur dioxide, which acts as a preservative. Blackstrap molasses is made from subsequent boiling, and although it has less sugar, it contains large amounts of micronutrients, including iron, calcium, magnesium, and potassium. It is commonly used as a diet supplement, as well as in cattle feed and large-scale food manufacturing. Molasses from sugar beets is a different product and is not marketed to the general public.

Corn Syrup

This sweet syrup is made from cornstarch. Similar to the way carbohydrates are broken down in your system, acids and enzymes when added to liquefied cornstarch turn it into glucose with a small amount of dextrose and maltose. Another enzyme is used to create high-fructose corn syrup. It is a complicated process, but even so, high-fructose corn syrup is cheaper to produce and transport than sugar. High-fructose corn syrup has the same level of sweetness as sugar, and because it is less expensive, it is used far more frequently in manufacturing food products. In fact, Americans now consume more high-fructose corn syrup than any other form of sugar.

Honey

In an effort to curb your intake of refined sugars, consider using honey as a sweetener. Twice as sweet as sucrose, honey has a unique flavor that enhances baked goods. It is rich in antioxidants, and long-term use has been shown to provide health benefits, including improved digestion, a stronger immune system, and lower cholesterol.

Date Sugar

Date sugar is another option. It contains nothing except ground dried dates, but it is equally as sweet as refined sugar. It has the added benefits of fiber, which slows down its absorption into your body, and all the vitamins and minerals of dates. It does not melt like sugar, so it's not good to use to sweeten coffee. But it is terrific in cakes and wherever you shake sugar for sweet crunchy toppings.

Maple Syrup

The majority of syrups in your market are made from corn syrup. But the real thing, made from reduced maple sap, is full of minerals and antioxidants. Lighter colored maple syrup is less concentrated than the dark stuff.

Agave Nectar

From the same plant that gives us tequila comes a syrup sweeter than cane sugar but with a very low glycemic index value, so it is absorbed more slowly into the bloodstream. This prevents it from raising blood sugar levels significantly, eliminating the highs and lows associated with sugar intake. For this reason, it's favored by people with diabetes and hypoglycemia. Creative chefs substitute agave nectar anywhere sugar or honey would ordinarily be used: barbecue sauces, marinades, baked goods, and so on. It adds a distinctive sweet flavor, reminiscent of tequila. Agave nectar is available through Internet sources (*www.rawagave.com*, *www.agavenectar.com*) and at health food stores.

Stevia

This sweetener is extracted from an herb (called stevia, sweetleaf, or sugarleaf) that is 300 times sweeter than granulated sugar but with a gylcemic index of zero. This means it will not affect your blood sugar level, producing no highs or lows. It doesn't melt or caramelize like sugar, but it dissolves nicely in liquids.

FACT

The glycemic index (GI) measures how fast food raises your blood sugar. Glucose, which raises your blood sugar most rapidly, has a GI of 100. Foods with high GI numbers are good for quickly raising blood sugar and when you want a burst of energy for intense exercise. Foods with low GI numbers are best to eat to support general activities or long periods of steady exertion.

Sugar Myths

Because sugar is such a beloved part of the American diet, it is no surprise that a few old wives' tales have sprung up around it.

Myth 1: Sugar Makes You Fat

The fact is that sugar is a part of a natural, healthy diet, and consumed as part of a well-balanced, natural diet, it will not cause excessive weight gain. Unfortunately, a well-balanced natural diet is not what most Americans consume. Most Americans eat a hefty amount of foods that contain added sugar. Added sugar is found in nearly all manufactured foods, including soda, juice, breads, condiments, cereals, and yogurts. These added sugars are considered the main contributor to the rise of obesity in America.

Myth 2: Sugar Is Addicting

Human DNA has a built-in craving for sweet food, but not for refined sugar. Primitive peoples needed to pad their bodies with excess weight for the long winter and times of famine, but they relied on sweet foods that were nutritious and nontoxic. We no longer have such needs, but we still experience the physiological desire for sweets. The key to combating this cruel side of evolution is to exercise some restraint. Get your sweet fix in as natural a form as you can and eat only enough to initially satisfy that sweet tooth.

Myth 3: A Healthy Diet Eliminates All Sugar

It would be unhealthy, and practically impossible, to eliminate all sugar from your diet. Sugar is a natural element in every kind of food, except meat. But eliminating the added sugars that do not naturally occur in foods is a great way to increase the nutritive values of your daily diet. Check labels regularly and opt for homemade over packaged foods to reduce your sugar intake.

Myth 4: White Sugar Is the Worst

Although it is true that white refined sugar is bad for you, it is no worse than brown sugar, "raw" sugar, powdered sugar, corn syrup, or any of the ingredients on food labels that end in "-ose." All refined sugars should be limited in favor of natural sugars. It is true that natural sugars break down in your body in the same way as refined sugars do, but it takes longer, and natural sugars provide additional nutrients.

Artificial Sweeteners

The Food and Drug Administration (FDA) has approved five artificial or "nonnutritive" sweeteners for human consumption. Testing is ongoing with all of these products, and their safety is still in question.

Saccharine

Used as an artificial sweetener for more than 100 years, saccharine is more than 200 times sweeter than sucrose, and it doesn't raise blood sugar levels. In the 1970s, it was found to cause cancer in rats and a ban was proposed. Because the effect has not been seen in humans, the product is still in use, but the labels must carry a warning. Saccharine is found in Sweet'N Low, Sweet Twin, and Necta Sweet.

Aspartame

This artificial sweetener is used in thousands of products all over the world. It contains 4 calories per gram, but it is about 200 times sweeter than sucrose, so you don't need much. A can of diet soda typically contains about 225 mg. There are many claims of adverse health effects from the ingestion of aspartame, including headaches, dizziness, anxiety, cramps, multiple sclerosis, lupus, and cancer. Headaches and depression have indeed been shown to occur in people with sensitivities who ingest aspartame. Aspartame isn't safe for people with a rare hereditary disease called phenylketonuria (PKU), and this is indicated on the label. Brain tumors have resulted in rats that ingest aspartame, but studies continue on the correlation between aspartame and human cancer. Dieters have also reported that aspartame increases appetite, especially cravings for carbohydrates. Aspartame is found in NutraSweet and Equal.

Acesulfame Potassium K

Two hundred times sweeter than sucrose, this product is generally used as a flavor enhancer and preservative. It contains the carcinogen methylene chloride, which, with long exposure, causes headaches, nausea, depression, liver and kidney disease, and cancer in humans. It has only undergone one initial testing. Acesulfame potassium K is found in Sunett and Sweet One.

Sucralose

This sweetener is 600 times sweeter than sucrose. It is the most recent addition to the list of artificial sweeteners and is currently used in nearly 5,000 products. Its big draw is that it can be used in baking, whereas other artificial sweeteners cannot. It has 391 calories per 110 grams, but because so little is needed, the amounts are small per serving and do not need to be reported on labels. The product is said to be made from sugar, but that is a bit misleading. Reports indicate it was discovered when scientists were treating sugar with a multitude of chemicals trying to create an insecticide. Adverse symptoms from sucralose consumption include gastrointestinal disorders, skin irritation, chest pain, anxiety, and depression. Sucralose is found in Splenda.

Neotame

This is a new sweeter version of aspartame, more than 7,000 times sweeter than sucrose. It was developed to be a version of aspartame that is safe for people with PKU. The FDA has given initial approval, but study continues. Neotame is used widely in food manufacturing.

Recipes

Strawberry Rhubarb Smoothie

This is a great way to eat fresh summer rhubarb, which combines well with strawberries. To use these ingredients as the basis for a sauce or pie filling, omit the liquid and blend the ingredients together.

INGREDIENTS | SERVES 2

3 small rhubarb stalks, chopped into pieces

2 cups strawberries, with green tops discarded

2 cups almond milk

1 teaspoon cinnamon

2 tablespoons organic honey

1 tablespoon maca root powder (optional)

Place all the ingredients into a blender and blend until smooth.

PER SERVING Calories: 367 • Fat: 22 g • Protein: 10 g • Sodium: 16 mg • Carbohydrates: 51 g • Fiber: 5 g

Mimosas with Fresh Mint and Oranges

This beverage is just the right thing for Sunday morning brunch.

INGREDIENTS | SERVES 2

1 orange

2 cups fresh orange juice

1 cup sparkling mineral water

4 fresh mint leaves, for garnish

Mimosa

These drinks are usually made with bubbly champagne. The sparkling mineral water gives the same light, refreshing effect without the alcohol.

1. Slice orange in half. Cut two thin slices of the orange (shaped like a wheel) and save them to use as a garnish.

2. Stir orange juice together with the sparkling water.

3. Serve in champagne flutes and garnish each glass with two mint leaves and one thin orange wheel slice.

PER SERVING Calories: 112 • Fat: 0 g • Protein: 2 g • Sodium: 4 mg • Carbohydrates: 15 g • Fiber: 0 g

Bloody Mary with Fresh Tomatoes and Spices

This is a delicious, nonalcoholic version of the popular cocktail.
Some optional garnishes include pickle spears or lemon slices.

INGREDIENTS | SERVES 2

5 large tomatoes
½ teaspoon fresh horseradish (optional)
1 teaspoon ground black pepper
½ teaspoon cayenne pepper powder
1 tablespoon lemon juice
1 teaspoon celery salt (optional)
2 cups ice
2 celery sticks
6 green olives

1. Juice tomatoes and horseradish, if using, and mix with black pepper, cayenne pepper, lemon juice, and salt (optional).

2. Fill 2 pint glasses with 1 cup of ice each and put 1 celery stick into each glass.

3. Fill pint glasses with tomato mixture and garnish with olives.

PER SERVING Calories: 110 • Fat: 2 g • Protein: 5 g • Sodium: 1,329 mg • Carbohydrates: 20 g • Fiber: 3 g

Mango Salsa

This sweeter version of salsa is good served with wraps and with Mexican pâté.
It can also be used as a dip with slices of vegetables such as cucumber, celery, or zucchini.

INGREDIENTS | SERVES 2

½ cup tomato, diced
1 cup fresh mango, seeded and diced
¼ cup white or red onion, diced
¼ cup diced cucumber
¼ teaspoon salt
½ tablespoon minced jalapeño pepper
1 tablespoon lime juice
2 tablespoons minced fresh cilantro

Stir all the ingredients together in a bowl and let the mixture sit for 10 minutes in the refrigerator to marinate.

PER SERVING Calories: 77 • Fat: 0 g • Protein: 1 g • Sodium: 296 mg • Carbohydrates: 17 g • Fiber: 3 g

Baba Ganoush

A good recipe to serve with falafel or tabouleh salad. Soaking the eggplant in salt water softens it and creates a texture similar to roasted eggplant. Another popular method for softening the eggplant is to slice it into thin strips, freeze it overnight, and then thaw.

INGREDIENTS | SERVES 4

2 cups eggplant, sliced thin

3 tablespoons lemon juice

2 tablespoons tahini

1 clove garlic, minced

1 teaspoon cumin

½ teaspoon black pepper

Salt, to taste

1 teaspoon paprika, for garnish

1 teaspoon olive oil, for garnish

2 tablespoons fresh chopped parsley, for garnish

Baba Ganoush

Baba ganoush is a popular Middle Eastern pâté and dip made from eggplant and spices. It is a wonderful complement to hummus and has a similar texture.

1. Place eggplant strips in a bowl or casserole dish and cover with 2 cups salt water. Add 1 teaspoon salt for every cup of water. Soften the eggplant by soaking it overnight in salt water in the refrigerator for 6–12 hours.

2. Drain the eggplant.

3. Place the eggplant, lemon juice, tahini, garlic, cumin, black pepper, and salt in a food processor with an S blade, and process until smooth.

4. Pour mixture into serving bowls, sprinkle on paprika, and drizzle a little olive oil on top. Garnish with fresh parsley.

PER SERVING Calories: 59 • Fat: 4 g • Protein: 2 g • Sodium: 8 mg • Carbohydrates: 5 g • Fiber: 2 g

Fruit Kebabs

The best fruit kebabs are made with fresh, seasonal fruit.
Try bananas, pineapples, melon, berries, peaches, grapes, and mango.
If your pickings are slim, use canned or frozen fruit, but not if it is packed in sugar syrup.

INGREDIENTS | SERVES 4

6–8 cups assorted seasonal fruits, cut into 1-inch chunks

6–8 wooden skewers

1 cup plain nonfat yogurt

Thread fruit on skewers in an alternating pattern. Serve with yogurt for dipping.

PER SERVING Calories: 180 • Fat: 1 g • Protein: 5 g • Sodium: 50 mg • Carbohydrates: 43 g • Fiber: 4 g

Morning Power Green Smoothie

Feel free to vary the fruit in this recipe, using frozen strawberries, blueberries, or banana. Add water to find the right consistency for your palate and adjust the sweetness to suit your taste.

INGREDIENTS | SERVES 1

1 cup vanilla-flavored hemp seed milk

½ cup frozen blueberries

1 tablespoon microplant powder of choice

1 tablespoon flaxseed meal

1 tablespoon hemp seed protein powder

Sweetener of choice, preferably stevia powder

1. Combine all ingredients in a blender and purée until smooth.

2. Serve immediately, while chilled and fresh, chewing well to better release the enzymes needed to digest the proteins, carbohydrates, and fats.

PER SERVING Calories: 242 • Fat: 13 g • Protein: 16 g • Sodium: 35 mg • Carbohydrates: 27 g • Fiber: 11 g

Kale Fennel Salad

Use a high-quality mayonnaise such as the Vegenaise brand found in natural-foods stores. Commercial brands are loaded with flavorings, colorings, and preservatives, plus refined sugar, which you want to avoid.

INGREDIENTS | SERVES 4

1 bunch fresh kale
1 bulb fresh fennel
1 teaspoon anchovy paste (or 3 anchovy fillets)
1 shallot
¼ cup extra-virgin olive oil
2 tablespoons balsamic vinegar
½ teaspoon garlic powder
1 teaspoon agave syrup
2 tablespoons mayonnaise
¼ cup toasted pumpkin seeds

A Low-Glycemic Sweetener

Agave syrup is made from the same cactus plant as tequila. It is a low-glycemic sweetener that won't spike your blood sugar. Use it in place of honey or maple syrup when sugar is called for in your recipes.

1. Wash and drain the kale. Run a sharp knife down the length of the stem to remove the leaf and set aside.

2. Cover the bottom of a large skillet with ½" of water; set kale into the pan. Cover, bring to a boil, reduce heat, and simmer until kale is tender but still bright green.

3. While kale is cooking, slice the fennel into narrow strips and set aside.

4. In a blender or using a mortar and pestle, combine anchovy, shallot, oil, vinegar, garlic, agave, and mayonnaise; mix to a dressing consistency.

5. Rinse cooked kale under cool water, drain, and press out water. Chop kale well; place in a medium-size salad bowl along with the fennel.

6. Spoon dressing over salad; toss well, or serve dressing on the side. Serve salad on individual plates.

7. Top with toasted pumpkin seeds before eating.

PER SERVING Calories: 280 • Fat: 21 g • Protein: 5 g • Sodium: 235 mg • Carbohydrates: 22 g • Fiber: 3 g

Aduki Fudge Brownies

Enjoy this healthy alternative to regular fudge brownies without spiking your blood sugar levels. Chestnuts provide balanced sweetness that is low in fat and high in complex carbohydrates. For a delicious treat, serve in a parfait topped with raspberry jam and almond crème.

INGREDIENTS | SERVES 12

1 cup cooked aduki beans
¾ cup roasted chestnuts
½ cup brown rice syrup
¼ cup raisins
1 tablespoon grain coffee
2 tablespoons almond butter
1 teaspoon vanilla extract
½ cup toasted almonds, chopped
1½ tablespoons agar flakes
¼ cup apple juice

1. Mix beans, chestnuts, rice syrup, and raisins in a large saucepan and cook over low heat for 5 minutes. Put mixture through a food mill or grind in a food processor until creamy.

2. Add grain coffee, almond butter, vanilla extract, and almonds.

3. In a large saucepan, mix agar flakes in apple juice and add aduki mixture. Cook over low heat for 10 minutes, stirring constantly

4. Pour into a cake pan and cool in refrigerator until set. Cut into bite-sized squares.

PER SERVING Calories: 161 • Fat: 5 g • Protein: 4 g • Sodium: 14 mg • Carbohydrate: 25 g • Fiber: 3 g

Lemon Millet Bars

Sour lemon acts as a tonic to the liver, stimulates bile production, and creates an alkalinizing effect in the body. Lemons are often used to used to lift people's spirits, calming anxiety and reducing depression.

INGREDIENTS | SERVES 12

¾ cup millet

5 cups apple juice

1 tablespoon brown rice syrup

Juice of 1 lemon

Zest of 1 lemon

Pinch of salt

3 tablespoons agar flakes

3 tablespoons kuzu

½ cup toasted almonds, ground, for garnish

Grated coconut, optional

Mint leaves, for garnish

Agar

Agar (also known as agar-agar) is a clear, odorless, tasteless sea vegetable used to gel kantens and desserts. Rich in calcium, agar helps counterbalance mineral loss from acidic sweeteners. Agar's cooling energy also relieves the heavy feeling after a meal. Because of its mild laxative effect, kanten is recommended for constipation.

1. Soak ¾ cup millet overnight in 2¼ cups apple juice. Bring to boil, lower heat, and simmer, covered, for 25 minutes.

2. Pour millet into a 9" × 9" baking pan and press down until millet covers the bottom of the pan.

3. In another saucepan, mix 2½ cups apple juice and remaining ingredients, except kuzu, ¼ cup apple juice, and garnishes. Bring to a boil, lower heat, and simmer, stirring until agar is dissolved. Dissolve kuzu in ¼ cup apple juice. Add kuzu mixture and simmer for 2 minutes. Pour mixture over millet crust and refrigerate until set, about 2 hours.

4. Slice into squares. Sprinkle ground almonds or grated coconut on top. Serve cold with mint leaves.

PER SERVING Calories: 125 • Fat: 3 g • Protein: 2.3 g • Sodium: 17 mg • Carbohydrate: 26 g • Fiber: 2 g

Blueberry Waffle Cakes

Nondairy milks such as rice, oat, almond, or soy milk work well with baked goods.
They are equivalent to a 2% dairy milk in consistency.

INGREDIENTS | MAKES 12 (4-INCH) PANCAKES OR WAFFLES

1 cup fresh or frozen blueberries
2 tablespoons spelt flour
2 cups spelt flour
1½ teaspoons baking soda
½ teaspoon salt
1 cup soy or rice milk (you may need to use a little more or less)
1 egg
1 tablespoon agave syrup
Plain yogurt, for garnish
Fresh blueberries, for garnish

1. Toss the blueberries in the 2 tablespoons of spelt flour; set aside.

2. Combine remaining ingredients (except syrup) in a blender; purée until smooth.

3. Pour batter into a bowl; gently stir in blueberries.

4. Pour ¼–⅓ cup batter onto heated waffle iron; cook until steam diminishes, about 1–2 minutes.

5. Remove to a plate; top with yogurt, agave syrup, and fresh blueberries.

PER PANCAKE OR WAFFLE Calories: 90 • Fat: 1.5 g • Protein: 4 g • Sodium: 12 mg • Carbohydrates: 16 g • Fiber: 3 g

Blueberry Cooking Time

When using fresh blueberries in batter, increase the cooking time. For the waffle recipe, wait an extra 1–2 minutes after the steam diminishes before removing the waffle. You may have to experiment with time depending on the size and temperature of your waffle iron.

Ginger Pear Wheat Pancakes

Add ¼ cup chopped walnuts to the chopped pears to give these pancakes a little texture and kick.

INGREDIENTS | SERVES 3

1½ cups whole-wheat flour
2 tablespoons applesauce
1 tablespoon brown sugar
1 cup water
1½ teaspoons baking powder
1½ teaspoons ground ginger
1 teaspoon ground cinnamon
2 chopped pears

1. Combine whole-wheat flour, applesauce, brown sugar, water, and baking powder in a medium bowl.

2. Add ginger and ground cinnamon.

3. Fold in the chopped pears.

4. Pour the batter onto a hot griddle or skillet, ¼ cup for each pancake, and cook until golden.

PER SERVING Calories: 267 • Fat: 1 g • Protein: 9 g • Sodium: 11 mg • Carbohydrates: 60 g • Fiber: 6.4 g

Poached Pears in Apple Cider

Poach autumn pears in spicy, sweet apple cider broth and reduce to make thick syrup. For variety, add apples and cranberries and purée to make spicy apple or cranberry sauce.

INGREDIENTS | SERVES 6

6 pears
2 quarts apple cider
1 stick cinnamon
1 teaspoon star anise
1 teaspoon cloves
1 tablespoon vanilla extract
2 slices fresh ginger
6 sprigs fresh mint leaves
Orange zest, for garnish

1. Cut pears in half and core. In a saucepan, add pears, cider, cinnamon, star anise, cloves, vanilla, and ginger. Bring to boil, lower heat, and simmer, covered, for 15–20 minutes or until pears are just tender.

2. Remove pears to a plate. Raise heat and bring cider mixture to boil. Cook until mixture is reduced to about 1½ cups of syrup. Strain and pour syrup over pears.

3. Garnish with the mint sprigs and orange zest.

PER SERVING Calories: 262 • Fat: 1 g • Protein: 1 g • Sodium: 15 mg • Carbohydrate: 65 g • Fiber: 6 g

Carrot Ginger Soup

Ginger adds dynamic energy to this soup. You can vary this recipe by adding winter squash, sweet potatoes, beets, or cashews. Adding almond or coconut milk softens the spicy edge of this soup.

INGREDIENTS | SERVES 5

1 cup onion, diced

2 clove garlic, crushed

1 teaspoon olive oil

4 medium carrots, diced

5 cups spring water

1½ teaspoon sweet white miso

¼ teaspoon ginger juice

¼ cup parsley, chopped

1. In a soup pot, sauté onion and garlic in olive oil until translucent.

2. Add carrots and water. Bring to boil, reduce heat, and simmer, covered, until carrots are soft, about 20 minutes.

3. Purée miso in a little cooking liquid. Add miso purée to soup.

4. Add ginger juice. Simmer 3 more minutes.

5. Purée soup in a food mill or blender. Garnish with parsley.

PER SERVING Calories: 47 • Fat: 1 g • Protein: 1 g • Sodium: 75 mg • Carbohydrate: 9 g • Fiber: 2 g

Carrot Onion Butter

Carrot onion butter is a kind of sweet vegetable jam used as a spread on toast, rice cakes, or muffins. Sauté 5 cups diced carrots and 5 cups diced onion in 2 tablespoons olive oil for 5 minutes. Add water to cover vegetables. Add a pinch sea salt, bring to boil, lower heat, and simmer, covered. After several hours, sweet vegetables will become thick jam.

CHAPTER 7

Fats and Oils

These essential nutrients are not "empty" calories in your diet. They not only flavor foods, they also provide a sense of fullness and are necessary in absorbing fat-soluble vitamins and minerals. This chapter explains how to manage fats and oils in your diet. Unfortunately, some fat sources are detrimental to your health. But if you equate "fat" with "bad," you're out of the loop, so let's reel you back in to the benefits of natural energy sources.

What Is Fat, and Why Do You Need It?

Fat is necessary for good health, but not in the quantities most Americans consume it. You need it to transport fat-soluble vitamins, insulate you in winter, and cushion falls or other types of impact to your body. For good health, however, it's important to understand and choose the right kind of fat.

Fat is a macronutrient, providing you with a concentrated source of energy and vital calories. The chemical name for this group of nutrients is lipids, and it includes fat, oil, and lecithin. Lipids are found in both plants and animals. In general, when stored at room temperature, fat is solid and oil is liquid.

ESSENTIAL

Lecithin is a natural emulsifying agent, which means it can help combine two ingredients that don't naturally combine, such as oil and water. The lecithin in an egg yolk is what lets you emulsify mayonnaise and thicken salad dressings. Soy-derived lecithin is used in hundreds of products, including chocolate.

Fatty Acids

Fatty acids are the building blocks of fat. They are linked together in long chains of carbon and hydrogen atoms. If a fatty acid chain is filled to capacity with hydrogen atoms, it is called saturated. This fat is thick, like butter.

If hydrogen is missing, it is called unsaturated. The amount of missing hydrogen determines whether the fat is monounsaturated or polyunsaturated. This type of fat is thin, as in oil.

All fat, including the fat you find in food, is made of a mixture of saturated and unsaturated fats. The majority of the fat a food contains determines its classification as saturated or unsaturated.

Fat is difficult for your body to digest and utilize because fat and water do not mix. Bile is the key to your utilization of fat. Made by the liver and secreted by the gallbladder, bile can break the triglycerides into their components—fatty acids and glycerol—for absorption.

Saturated Fats

This type of fat is found mainly in animal-based foods. It can easily be identified, because the foods are solid at room temperature. You'll find saturated fat in meat, butter, cheese, and lard.

These are the most dangerous types of fat because they appear to raise blood cholesterol levels. They may inhibit the liver's ability to clear out low-density lipoproteins (LDL) and actually stimulate their production. The result is an increased likelihood of atherosclerosis and coronary artery disease.

Saturated fats are seldom found in plants. The exceptions are palm oil and coconut oil. These plants contain a large amount of saturated fatty acids, which are solid at room temperature. They are free of trans fat, and as such are often encouraged for use in place of hydrogenated oils. Additionally, they are easier for your body to absorb than trans fat.

Unsaturated Fats

These fats are liquid at room temperature. Generally referred to as oils, they come mainly from plant sources. These fats have a short shelf life, and are likely to spoil.

There are two types of unsaturated fats: monounsaturated and polyunsaturated. Monounsaturated fats occur in olive, canola, and nut oils, including peanut oil. Polyunsaturated fats include plant oils such as safflower, sunflower, cottonseed, sesame, corn, and soybean. Unsaturated fats have been shown to actually lower the low-density lipoproteins (LDL) in your blood.

The only animal oil that is not saturated is polyunsaturated fish oil. These oils contain healthy omega-3 fatty acids and are an essential part of a healthy diet. If you do not eat fish at least twice a week, it's a good idea to take fish oil supplements to ensure you're getting your omega-3s.

FACT

When fat spoils it is called rancid. Oxygen and light are the main culprits in shortening fat's shelf life. Foods that contain fat should be refrigerated if intended for long-term use.

Trans Fat

This is the worst kind of fat. Trans fat has been shown to both lower the good cholesterol in your body and raise the bad. Not a healthy prospect. To make matters worse, in recent years trans fats have been used extensively in manufactured foods.

To make hydrogenated fat, extra hydrogen is added to unsaturated vegetable fat. Trans fats and partially hydrogenated fats are listed on labels.

Because trans fats are artificially saturated, the molecular chains are not straight like natural saturated fats, so they do not line up and pack together tightly. You can see this by comparing the way butter (which has no trans fat) and margarine (which is pure trans fat) spread when chilled.

What Is Cholesterol?

Cholesterol is a type of lipid found in the cells of all body tissues. It is not considered essential because your body makes it in the liver. It is a fatty substance, but unlike fat, it does not provide you with energy. You can't taste it or smell it, but it is in the food you eat, and your body needs it to function properly.

Every cell in your body contains cholesterol. Cholesterol carried in your bloodstream is called blood serum cholesterol. It is transported by blood plasma throughout the body and is used to make cell membranes, bile acids that allow us to digest fats, hormones, and vitamin D. Like so many things, too much cholesterol can be dangerous.

When it is in your food it is called dietary cholesterol. Found mainly in animals, you get lots of it in shrimp, egg yolks, dairy products, and meat.

LDL and HDL

Because fat does not dissolve in water, it is transported through the bloodstream by water-soluble proteins called lipoproteins. They wrap the cholesterol and triglycerides like a package and deliver it throughout the body. From the liver, triglycerides and cholesterol are secreted into plasma, where they are joined with low-density lipoprotein (LDL).

Termed the "bad cholesterol," LDL is thought to increase the risk of heart disease, heart attacks, and stroke. Healthy blood has fairly few large particles of LDL. If too many accumulate, problems occur. When LDL accumulates on the walls of the arteries it can harden them and cause blockage. This is called arterial plaque. If blockage occurs in a main heart artery, a heart attack is the result. If blockage occurs in a major brain artery, stroke can result.

High-density lipoproteins (HDL) circulate in the blood, picking up cholesterol and excess plaque and transporting it back to the liver, where it is excreted as bile. For optimal health, levels of LDL should be low, and levels of HDL should be high. Your cholesterol levels can be determined by a blood test. Healthy ratios of total cholesterol to HDL should be below 5:1.

Lowering Your Cholesterol Level

Cholesterol is measured in milligrams per deciliter of blood (mg/dl). When measuring LDL, 130 milligrams per deciliter is considered good, 160 is high. If you have heart disease, your target is 70 mg/dl.

In women, the target level range for HDL is 50–60 milligrams per deciliter. Men should aim for 40–50. Lower levels are considered risky.

When planning your diet, keep your saturated fat intake low. It should never constitute more than 10 percent of your total fat intake.

Polyunsaturated Fatty Acids: The Omegas

Omega-3 and omega-6 are essential fatty acids, which means you need them for good health, but your body cannot manufacture them. The name of these acids is an indication of where along the fatty acid chain (the "E" tail) hydrogen atoms are missing.

FACT

Flaxseeds are primarily used to make linseed oil, but they are also marketed in health food stores. Look for them near the grains, and add them to pilafs, salads, cereals, and breads.

Omega-3 is found in fish oil and plant oils, especially flaxseed oil. It is believed to reduce inflammation, improve blood circulation, and decrease the thickness of arterial walls, a significant benefit to people with high blood serum cholesterol. Omega-6 is found in nuts, whole grains, legumes, sesame oil, and soy oil. When used together to replace saturated fats, these fatty acids can reduce high blood pressure and cholesterol.

Cooking with Fats

Fats are an important part of cuisine. They carry flavor throughout a recipe, and bind and emulsify ingredients. The key to healthy cooking is knowing which fats to use.

▼ **Specific Fat Content of Commonly Used Oils**

Oil	Saturated Fat	Polyunsaturated Fat	Monounsaturated Fat
Canola Oil	7%	32% (21% omega-6, 11% omega-3)	61%
Coconut Oil	91%	2% (2% omega-6)	7%
Corn Oil	13%	58% (57% omega-6, 1% omega-3)	29%
Flaxseed Oil	9%	73% (16% omega-6, 57% omega-3)	18%
Olive Oil	15%	10% (9% omega-6, 1% omega-3)	75%
Safflower Oil	8%	15% (15% omega-6, 1% omega-3)	77%
Sunflower Oil	12%	72% (71% omega-6, 1% omega-3)	16%

Oils

Oil is an essential part of a salad. Without oil, the dressing would slip off the lettuce and pool at the bottom of the bowl. Just think about the way oil feels when it gets on your hands. Oil spreads flavor throughout a recipe like it spreads on your hands. You need it in recipes, but you don't need much.

Whenever possible, use mainly monounsaturated oils, which contribute to high-density lipoproteins. Olive and peanut oils are good choices. They have fairly distinctive flavors and can easily overpower a dish, so use a light hand. If a neutral oil is called for, canola is a good monounsaturated choice.

Fats

Like oil, fats are added to recipes to tenderize, moisten, and prolong shelf life. Because fats change their consistency when heated, the temperature indicated in the recipe is important.

The most frequent fat used for baking is butter. Unsalted butter is preferred by most bakers and chefs for its superior flavor. The lack of salt also gives the cook control over the amount of salt in a recipe. Salted butter can always be detected, as it makes the dish saltier than necessary. If you have no choice but to use salted butter, you should omit or reduce the amount of salt in the recipe.

FACT

The USDA suggests that you consume no more than 7 teaspoons of fat and oil each day. This includes not just the added butter on your baked potato but also the fats and oils found naturally in foods as well as those added to prepared foods.

Margarine is never a good choice. Its flavor is inferior, and because it is typically a trans fat, it is an unhealthy food. Also, its higher melting point leaves behind an unpleasant aftertaste. Because vegetable fats do not melt at body temperatures, as animal fats do, margarine coats the tongue and lingers on the palate long after the food is swallowed.

Butter, although a saturated animal-based fat, is preferable to margarine in maintaining a healthy diet. However, problems occur with any saturated fats when eaten in excess, so consume butter (and all fats) in moderation.

Like butter, lard is preferable to margarine. Lard is less popular today than in the past, but it is often preferred by bakers, especially for pie dough. It creates a superior flakiness that cannot be achieved with butter or shortening, and because it is an animal product, it leaves behind no unpleasant aftertaste. It is generally rendered from pork, although in other parts of the world it is made from other animal fats, too.

Recipes

Creamy Garlic Soup

The shiitake mushrooms in this dish add a distinctive flavor to the stock. Once they have soaked, you can slice them and use them later in a stir-fry or omelet.

INGREDIENTS | SERVES 6

4 heads of garlic
6 cups chicken or vegetable stock
4 dried shiitake mushrooms
1 teaspoon sea salt
14 ounces silken tofu
6 teaspoons extra-virgin olive oil
¼ cup parsley, minced
¼ cup pine nuts, toasted

Quick Garlic Bread

Slice a piece of sourdough bread and rub the top with a slice of garlic clove. Then brush the bread with olive oil and top with grated Romano cheese. Run under the broiler until golden brown and serve alongside the soup. Add a simple green salad to balance out the meal.

1. Preheat oven to 375°F.

2. Wrap garlic in aluminum foil; bake 20 minutes, or until tender.

3. In a large saucepan, add stock and shiitake mushrooms; simmer gently while garlic is baking.

4. Remove garlic from oven, cool, remove aluminum foil, and slice off flat end of garlic head. Squeeze softened cloves into a bowl; set aside.

5. In a blender, purée roasted garlic, salt, silken tofu, and 2 cups stock until smooth.

6. Remove shiitake mushrooms from stock and set aside to use at another time. Add puréed tofu mixture to the stock; heat just until warmed through.

7. Ladle soup into individual bowls; drizzle a teaspoon of olive oil along surface. Top with minced parsley and toasted pine nuts.

PER SERVING Calories: 270 • Fat: 11 g • Protein: 10 g • Sodium: 364 mg • Carbohydrates: 36 g • Fiber: 3 g

Turkey Shish Kebabs

You can make this excellent dish with cubed chicken if you prefer.
Serve with a gelatin salad and some breadsticks.

INGREDIENTS | SERVES 6

1¼ pounds turkey tenderloin

⅓ cup chili sauce

2 tablespoons lemon juice

1 tablespoon brown sugar

12 mushrooms

12 cherry tomatoes

1 zucchini, sliced ½-inch thick

1 green bell pepper, sliced

2 red onions, quartered

2 tablespoons olive oil

1. Cut turkey into 1½-inch cubes and place in a bowl. In a small bowl, stir together the chili sauce, lemon juice, and brown sugar. Pour over the turkey cubes and toss to coat. Cover and refrigerate for 4–8 hours, stirring occasionally.

2. When ready to eat, prepare and preheat grill. Remove turkey from marinade, reserving marinade. Thread turkey onto metal skewers alternately with mushrooms, cherry tomatoes, zucchini, bell pepper, and onions.

3. Brush lightly with oil and place on grill rack about 6 inches above medium-hot coals. Grill, turning occasionally, and basting frequently with the reserved marinade, until the turkey is cooked through and the vegetables are tender, about 9–10 minutes.

PER SERVING Calories: 291.51 • Fat: 10.34 grams • Protein: 16 g • Sodium: 281.65 mg • Carbohydrates: 10 g • Fiber: 1 g

Cottage Pie with Carrots, Parsnips, and Celery

Cottage pie is similar to the more familiar shepherd's pie, but it's made with beef instead of lamb. This version uses lots of vegetables and lean meat.

INGREDIENTS | SERVES 6

1 large onion, diced

3 cloves garlic, minced

1 carrot, diced

1 parsnip, diced

1 stalk celery, diced

1 pound 94% lean ground beef

1½ cups beef stock

½ teaspoon hot paprika

½ teaspoon crushed rosemary

1 tablespoon Worcestershire sauce

½ teaspoon dried savory

⅛ teaspoon salt

¼ teaspoon freshly ground black pepper

1 tablespoon cornstarch and 1 tablespoon water, mixed (if necessary)

¼ cup minced fresh parsley

2¾ cups plain mashed potatoes

Save Time in the Morning

The night before cooking this dish, take a few minutes to cut up vegetables you'll need for the recipe. Place them in an airtight container or plastic bag and refrigerate until morning. Measure out dried spices and place them in a small container on the counter until needed.

1. Sauté the onions, garlic, carrots, parsnips, celery, and beef in a large nonstick skillet until the ground beef is browned. Drain off any excess fat and discard it. Place the mixture into a round 4-quart slow cooker. Add the stock, paprika, rosemary, Worcestershire sauce, savory, salt, and pepper. Stir.

2. Cook on low for 6–8 hours. If the meat mixture still looks very wet, create a slurry by mixing together 1 tablespoon cornstarch and 1 tablespoon water. Stir this into the meat mixture.

3. In a medium bowl, mash the parsley and potatoes using a potato masher. Spread on top of the ground beef mixture in the slow cooker. Cover and cook on high for 30–60 minutes or until the potatoes are warmed through.

PER SERVING Calories: 240 • Fat: 6 g • Protein: 20 g • Sodium: 420 mg • Carbohydrates: 26 g • Fiber: 2 g

Spiced Almond Falafels

This recipe is delicious served with pasta dishes and with salads.
These falafels are dehydrated and have a texture similar to cooked falafels.

INGREDIENTS | SERVES 4

2 cups almonds, soaked
1 garlic clove
2 tablespoons lemon juice
1 tablespoon sage
¼ teaspoon cayenne pepper powder
2 tablespoons liquid coconut oil

1. Using a food processor with an S blade, process all the ingredients together.

2. Form into little balls and dehydrate at 145°F for 2 hours. Turn down the temperature and continue dehydrating at 115°F for 12 hours.

PER SERVING Calories: 474 • Fat: 42 g • Protein: 15 g • Sodium: 1 mg • Carbohydrates: 9 g • Fiber: 9 g

Heated Oils

Research shows that deep-fried foods clog the arteries and contain carcinogens. This recipe will give you all the flavor of deep-fried falafel without the unhealthy fats.

Wild Rice–Stuffed Turkey Breast Cutlets

All this hearty dish needs is a side of steamed vegetables to make it a complete meal.

INGREDIENTS | SERVES 4

1 onion, sliced
4 ounces button mushrooms, minced
1 cup cooked wild rice
4 turkey breast cutlets (about 1 pound)
½ cup chicken or turkey stock

1. Place the onions and mushrooms on the bottom of a 4-quart slow cooker.

2. Divide the wild rice into four portions. Place a single portion in the center of each cutlet. Roll, rice-side in, and secure with a toothpick or kitchen twine. Place on top of the onions and mushrooms. Pour the broth over top.

3. Cook on low for 4 hours.

PER SERVING Calories: 190 • Fat: 1 g • Protein: 31 g • Sodium: 150 mg • Carbohydrates: 12 g • Fiber: 1 g

Orange Sesame Dressing

Citrus juices like orange, lemon, or lime balance heavy, oily foods and support liver function. Serve citrusy Orange Sesame Dressing over fish, hijiki sauté, or black japonica or forbidden rice.

INGREDIENTS | SERVES 4

1 tablespoon black or tan sesame seeds, toasted

1 tablespoon lemon juice

1 tablespoon sesame oil

1 tablespoon shoyu (soy sauce)

2 tablespoons orange juice

1 clove roasted garlic, optional

Ginger juice, optional

Grind sesame seeds in a suribachi bowl or food processor to make a paste. Add remaining ingredients and grind together.

PER SERVING Calories: 50 • Fat: 5 g • Protein: 1 g • Sodium: 226 mg • Carbohydrate: 2 g • Fiber: 0 g

Homemade Guacamole

Avocados are a unique fruit because they are naturally high in fat. Because you need some fat in your diet, guacamole is a healthy choice.

INGREDIENTS | SERVES 4

2 ripe avocados, peeled and seeded

½ cup tomatoes, diced

½ teaspoon fresh garlic, minced

½ teaspoon salt

1 teaspoon green chili, finely minced

1 teaspoon freshly squeezed lemon juice

½ cup fat-free sour cream

Mix all ingredients to desired texture.

PER SERVING Calories: 187 • Fat: 15 g • Protein: 4 g • Sodium: 300 mg • Carbohydrates: 12 g • Fiber: 3 g

Broccoli and Tomatoes in Anchovy Sauce

*Broccoli and tomatoes can be tossed with the sauce and served as a side dish.
Or, the whole recipe can be combined with cooked angel-hair pasta and served as
an entrée with a fresh green salad and a hunk of country whole-grain bread.*

INGREDIENTS | SERVES 4

⅓ cup extra-virgin olive oil

3 cloves garlic

6 anchovy fillets or 2 tablespoons anchovy paste

½ cup fresh parsley, stems removed

1 pound broccoli florets

2 large, ripe tomatoes

½ cup grated Romano cheese

Sea salt, to taste

What Does Water Sauté Mean?

When you want a quick, fat-free way to cook vegetables, while still retaining flavor and nutrients, a water sauté is the way to go. Simply pour 1–2 inches of water into a skillet, add the chopped vegetables, cover, and bring to a low simmer. Cook until the vegetables are just tender, then cool under running water and set aside until ready to use.

1. With a mortar and pestle or food processor, combine the oil, garlic, anchovies, and parsley; process to a loose paste. Add more oil as needed to get the right consistency.

2. Steam or water sauté the broccoli until just tender. Remove from heat; place in a medium-size bowl.

3. Quarter and chop tomatoes; add to the broccoli.

4. Spoon anchovy sauce into the broccoli and tomatoes; toss gently to coat.

5. Sprinkle with Romano cheese, add salt as desired, and serve.

PER SERVING Calories: 260 • Fat: 21 g • Protein: 8 g • Sodium: 187 g • Carbohydrates: 12 g • Fiber: 5 g

Spicy Mung Beans in Coconut Milk

Mung beans are often sprouted and used in salads or to top off Asian-style stir-fries. Traditionally, they are cooked in India, similarly to this recipe, where the dish is called a moong dhal. You don't need to presoak these beans, as they cook quickly and are easy to digest.

INGREDIENTS | SERVES 8

1 cup mung beans

4 cups water

1 onion

3 cloves garlic

1 hot pepper or 1 teaspoon red pepper flakes

2-inch piece fresh ginger

1 tablespoon coconut oil

1 tablespoon ghee (clarified butter)

1 teaspoon curry powder

1 teaspoon garam masala (Indian spices)

2 medium tomatoes

5½ ounces coconut milk

½ teaspoon sea salt

Clarified Butter

Clarified butter is regular butter that has had the milk solids and water removed, leaving behind a pure, golden-yellow butterfat. Also known as drawn butter, or ghee, it has a rich butter flavor with a shelf life of several months and a much higher smoke point than most oils. You can buy it ready-made in an Indian or natural foods market.

1. Wash and sort through the mung beans, removing any stones or other debris. In a large saucepan or Dutch oven, bring the mung beans and water to a boil over medium-high heat; cover, reduce, and allow to simmer until beans become tender, about 15 minutes.

2. Meanwhile, chop onion; mince garlic and pepper; and peel and mince ginger.

3. Heat oil and ghee in a skillet; sauté vegetables over medium-low heat, stirring from time to time, until onions are tender, about 4 minutes. Add curry powder and garam masala; stir well. Cook until spices release their aroma, about 1–2 minutes.

4. While onion-spice mixture is cooking, chop tomatoes; place in a blender or food processor and purée until smooth and liquid.

5. Pour tomatoes into mung beans along with onion-spice mixture. Add a small amount of water to skillet to "wash" out any remaining oil or spice adhering to the bottom of the pan; add to mung beans. Add coconut milk and salt to taste; stir well.

6. Reduce heat to simmer, cover, and cook another 30 minutes, or until beans have broken apart and flavors are well combined. (At this point, you could place the mung-bean mixture into a heated slow cooker and cook on low for a few hours until ready to serve.)

PER SERVING Calories: 170 • Fat: 8 g • Protein: 7 g • Sodium: 197 mg • Carbohydrates: 20 g • Fiber: 5 g

Lentil Walnut Pâté

Walnuts contain lots of monousaturated fats, which are important for good health

INGREDIENTS | SERVES 8

½ cup walnuts
2 green onions
1½ cups cooked lentils
¾ cup cooked brown rice
3 tablespoons tamari soy sauce
¾ cup rolled oats
2 tablespoons almond butter

What to Do with Walnuts

Walnuts can be served roasted as an appetizer or coated with melted butter and honey as a sweet, crunchy treat.

1. Preheat oven to 375°F.

2. Chop walnuts and green onions in food processor.

3. Combine remaining ingredients in food processor; process until smooth.

4. Spoon into a lightly oiled 8" × 8" baking pan; bake for 30 minutes.

5. Cool and serve with crackers, rice cakes, or as a sandwich spread.

PER SERVING Calories: 180 • Fat: 8 g • Protein: 7 g • Sodium: 378 mg • Carbohydrates: 20 g • Fiber: 6 g

Tempeh "Chicken" Salad

Turn this great dish into a sandwich, or slice up some tomatoes and serve on a bed of lettuce.

INGREDIENTS | SERVES 3–4

1 package tempeh, diced small
3 tablespoons vegan mayonnaise
2 teaspoons lemon juice
½ teaspoon garlic powder
1 teaspoon Dijon mustard
2 tablespoons sweet pickle relish
½ cup green peas
2 stalks celery, diced small
1 tablespoon chopped fresh dill (optional)

1. Cover tempeh with water and simmer for 10 minutes, until tempeh is soft. Drain and allow to cool completely.

2. Whisk together mayonnaise, lemon juice, garlic powder, mustard, and relish.

3. Combine tempeh, mayonnaise mixture, peas, celery, and dill, and gently toss to combine.

4. Chill for at least 1 hour before serving to allow flavors to combine.

PER SERVING Calories: 237 • Fat: 14 g • Protein: 16 g • Sodium: 233 mg • Carbohydrates: 21 g • Fiber: 2 g

Vegan Tzatziki

Use a vegan soy yogurt to make this classic Greek dip, which is best served very cold. A nondairy sour cream may be used instead of the soy yogurt, if you prefer.

INGREDIENTS | YIELDS 1½ CUPS

1½ cups vegan soy yogurt, plain or lemon flavored

1 tablespoon olive oil

1 tablespoon lemon juice

4 cloves garlic, minced

2 cucumbers, grated or chopped fine

1 tablespoon chopped fresh mint or fresh dill

1. Whisk together yogurt with olive oil and lemon juice until well combined.

2. Combine with remaining ingredients.

3. Chill for at least 1 hour before serving to allow flavors to mingle. Serve cold.

PER ¼ CUP: CALORIES 76 • Fat: 3 g • Protein: 2 g • Sodium: 10 mg • Carbohydrates: 10 g • Fiber: 1 g

What Is Tzatziki?

Tzatziki is a Greek appetizer. It consists of strained yogurt (usually made from sheep's milk or goat's milk) with cucumbers, garlic, salt, olive oil, and pepper.

Toad in a Hole

In Britain, Toad in a Hole involves baking sausages and Yorkshire pudding in a large pan with bacon fat drippings and flour. But this recipe—a Pennsylvania Dutch favorite—is far simpler and less fattening as well.

INGREDIENTS | SERVES 2

1 slice bread, any kind

Nonfat cooking spray

1 egg

Salt and pepper, to taste

1. Use a circular cookie cutter to cut a hole in the center of a slice of bread.

2. Place bread on a warm skillet that you've sprayed lightly with nonfat cooking spray.

3. Crack the egg and put it in the hole in the bread.

4. Fry and flip to desired consistency.

5. Season with salt and pepper to taste.

PER SERVING Calories: 72 • Fat: 3 g • Protein: 5 g • Sodium: 151 mg • Carbohydrates: 7 g • Fiber: 3 g

Flipping Toads

As it cooks, the egg adheres to the bread. This makes it super simple to flip the bread in the pan without worrying about dislodging the egg. Be sure to flip your eggs after they've had time to set. Otherwise, you risk getting runny egg all over the place, which won't affect taste but will leave you with a mess.

Grilled Tuna Niçoise

You can prepare the topping to this dish up to a day in advance.
The added time will intensify the flavors. Remember, when cooking fish of any kind, follow the ten-minutes-per-inch rule: ten minutes of moderate heat for every inch of thickness.

INGREDIENTS | SERVES 4

2 cups kalamata olives, pitted and halved

1 yellow onion, minced

¼ cup capers

2 tomatoes, chopped

¼ cup fresh parsley, chopped

½ cup olive oil

½ cup red wine vinegar

4 (3-ounce) tuna steaks

½ cup lemon juice

⅛ teaspoon kosher salt

½ teaspoon black pepper

1. Preheat grill on high heat. In a large bowl combine olives, onions, capers, tomatoes, parsley, olive oil, and wine vinegar. Toss together and set aside at room temperature.

2. Coat tuna steaks with lemon juice, salt, pepper, and grill. Cook 5–10 minutes per side, until meat is firm and cooked through. Serve immediately topped with olive mixture.

PER SERVING Calories: 565 • Fat: 47 g • Protein: 22 g • Sodium: 1,295 mg • Carbohydrates: 16 g • Fiber: 3 g

Sausage and Mushroom Omelet

If you like a little spice, add a dash of Tabasco sauce to kick up the flavor of this dish.

INGREDIENTS | SERVES 2

4 large egg whites

1 large whole egg

¼ teaspoon salt

1 tablespoon olive oil

½ cup chopped cooked turkey sausage

½ cup chopped mushrooms

1. Beat the egg whites and egg in a bowl. Mix in the salt.

2. Heat the olive oil in a small skillet on low heat.

3. Pour the egg mixture in the skillet to coat the surface. Cook until edges show firmness.

4. Add the sausage and mushrooms so they cover the entire mixture evenly. Fold one side over the other.

5. Flip the half-moon omelet so both sides are evenly cooked.

PER SERVING Calories: 266 • Fat: 20 g • Protein: 20 g • Sodium: 631 mg • Carbohydrates: 2.5 g • Fiber: 0.34 g

CHAPTER 8

All about Vitamins and Minerals

The sources of vitamins and minerals can be confusing when choosing between fruits, vegetables, grains, proteins, dairy, fortified foods, and supplements. All vitamin and mineral amounts vary, so you must consume a variety of foods to maintain balanced nutrition. It's best to stay as close as you can to the mainstream of natural foods in order to meet your vitamin and mineral needs. Unfortunately, the modern individual's diet doesn't always provide the correct amount of vitamins and minerals she needs for optimal health and so some basic supplementation is often beneficial.

The Importance of Daily Vitamin Intake

Vitamins are a necessary component of a healthy diet. They are considered essential nutrients because our bodies either do not make them, or do not make enough of them. They are essential for normal body functions—cell growth, blood cell production, hormone and enzyme synthesis, energy metabolism, and proper functioning of body systems, including the immune system, nervous system, circulatory system, and reproductive system.

Because no single food contains all the vitamins you need, you must obtain them through a variety of foods. You can take a pill that contains vitamins, but it is always preferable to get them the natural way. The reason is twofold. If you take a supplement because you assume your diet is poor, you may not be supplementing the right nutrients. More importantly, getting your vitamins by eating healthy foods provides the body with many other nutrients necessary for good health, including fiber, carbohydrates, protein, and water.

Fat-Soluble Vitamins

Four of the essential vitamins are fat soluble. That means that they dissolve in fat, not water, and are stored in the body's fatty tissue and in the liver. Because they can be stored for long periods of time, people consuming a well-balanced diet do not need to supplement them. In fact, because these vitamins hang around for quite a while, they are more prone to toxicity than the water-soluble vitamins.

A normal amount of fat in the diet is necessary to metabolize these fat-soluble vitamins. They are absorbed through the large intestine, and there must be some fat present for successful absorption. After absorption, these vitamins are stored in the liver until needed.

Vitamin A

Also known as retinol, vitamin A is primarily found in animal foods, including dairy products, fish, liver, and egg yolks. It has a pro-vitamin, called beta-carotene, which is found in vegetables with orange pigment, such as carrots, sweet potatoes, and apricots, as well as some dark, leafy greens including spinach and kale.

As you may have guessed by its aka "beta-carotene" and its presence in carrots, vitamin A is important for the health of your eyes. It is vital for night vision and the adjustments the eye regularly makes to various light levels. Vitamin A also helps keep skin healthy, promotes healthy bone and tooth growth, and is vital for proper cell division and reproduction. It strengthens and moistens mucous membranes, too, which helps you resist infections.

ESSENTIAL

A pro-vitamin is not a vitamin that has renounced its amateur status. Also known as a vitamin precursor, pro-vitamins are organic compounds that, once ingested, the body converts into a vitamin.

Deficiencies are rare, but symptoms may include night blindness and seriously dry and itchy skin, as well as slow tooth and bone growth. Signs of vitamin A toxicity include dry itchy skin, nausea, and headache. Excessive amounts of beta-carotene in the body may turn skin a pale orange.

Vitamin D

Because it is naturally synthesized by sunlight on your skin, vitamin D is sometimes called the sunshine vitamin. Ten minutes in the sun is enough to give you your daily dose. During the Industrial Revolution, when people began spending more time indoors, and the skies were clouded by pollutants, rickets was rampant. Rickets is a disease in which bones do not harden properly. Scientists suspected a dietary deficiency along the same lines as scurvy, and soon found that cod liver oil eliminated the disease. It was also noted that large doses of sunshine were restorative.

Vitamin D's main function is to control the absorption of calcium, which promotes the hardening of bones and teeth. Vitamin D deficiency leads to rickets in children, and a similar affliction in adults, known as osteomalacia. It might also be a contributor to osteoporosis. These conditions occur when bone mineralization is impaired, keeping bones from hardening properly. As a result, they become soft, weak, painful, and fragile. People who are exposed to minimal sunshine, who live in areas with lots of cloud or fog cover, spend much of their time indoors, or cover themselves with sunblock, are likely candidates for vitamin D deficiency.

Because of this, vitamin D has been added to many products, most notably milk. Small amounts occur naturally in a few foods, including sardines, herring, and cod liver oil.

Toxicity of vitamin D in mild forms leads to nausea, irritability, and weight loss. Severe cases result in mental and physical growth retardation, calcium in the blood, and kidney damage.

QUESTION

Will sunblock prevent vitamin D absorption?
Proper use of sunblock, with a sun protection factor (SPF) of 15, will deflect or absorb all but 7 percent of the UVB rays that synthesize vitamin D (and cause skin cancer). But most people fail to apply sunblock properly. You need at least an ounce, or about two tablespoons, and it should be applied fifteen to twenty minutes before going outdoors so that it has ample time to penetrate. Most people apply it too late, and too sparingly, cutting its effectiveness in half. Chances are you're still getting your vitamin D.

Vitamin E

This vitamin is a powerful antioxidant. Additionally, it works to protect vitamins A and C and red and white blood cells, promotes iron metabolism, and helps maintain nervous system tissue. Some past studies suggested that vitamin E can slow the development of heart disease, but current wisdom notes that diets high in all antioxidants lower risks of cancer and coronary disease. You'll find vitamin E in seeds, whole grains, and nuts.

Deficiency in vitamin E is rare, but toxicity can occur. Symptoms include nausea and gastrointestinal disorders.

Vitamin K

This vitamin is sometimes called the Band-Aid vitamin because its primary function is to aid in the clotting of blood. In fact, the K comes from the Danish word *koagulation*. Vitamin K also helps hold calcium in your bones. Naturally produced by bacteria in the intestines, it can also be found in dark, leafy green vegetables, including turnip greens, spinach, broccoli, and cabbage.

Deficiency results in excessive bleeding. Because vitamin K is formed by bacteria in the intestines, bacteria-killing antibiotics can interfere with its production. Also, because it is fat soluble, people who have difficulties digesting fat may become deficient in this vitamin.

ESSENTIAL

Antioxidants can slow, prevent, and reverse damage done by oxidation. Oxidation is an electron transfer process (the loss of electrons by a molecule, atom, or ion), which can produce free radicals. Free radicals damage body cells and tissues.

Water-Soluble Vitamins

Water-soluble vitamins dissolve in water, and, because your body is made mostly of water, they cannot be stored. Once ingested, they are quickly flushed out of your body through sweat and urine. In food, they are easily lost as a result of poor storage or excessive cooking. Therefore, you need a continuous supply of these vitamins to stay healthy.

Institutional food is likely to be deficient in water-soluble vitamins. Preparing food in large quantities frequently results in overcooked and reheated foods, which causes considerable loss of these nutrients.

Eight of the water-soluble vitamins were once thought to be the same compound, designated by early scientists as vitamin B. Later, they were shown to be several compounds and broken up into a group commonly known as the B complex. Cooking vegetables in water is the best way to eliminate water-soluble vitamins. Unless you are making soup, and therefore plan to consume the cooking liquid, you should steam or quickly sauté your veggies over high heat. Canned vegetables, which are subjected to high heat in the canning process, are short on B vitamins, too.

B1/Thiamin

The main function of thiamin is to create an enzyme (thiamin pyrophosphate) that is essential in the conversion of food to energy. It also contributes to the proper functioning of the nervous system by keeping the heart muscle elastic. Thiamin is found in whole grains, seeds, legumes, pork, and liver, and is fortified in many food products.

B2/Riboflavin

This vitamin's most important job is cell respiration. Oxygen and food molecules enter a cell, where enzymes release the food's and oxygen's energy. These enzymes contain riboflavin. If riboflavin is absent, the cells cannot release enough energy.

ESSENTIAL

Serious athletes, who are regularly expending a lot of energy, may benefit from increased riboflavin, due to its role in protein synthesis and energy metabolism.

Riboflavin also regulates cell growth, aids in the production of red blood cells, and is important for healthy hair and skin. It helps the immune system by making antibodies and keeping mucous membranes healthy and able to fight off germs. Some studies suggest that it can be useful in reducing migraine headaches.

Riboflavin is found in dark green vegetables and whole grains. It is also present in milk products, especially cottage cheese and yogurt. Because riboflavin is easily destroyed by light, packages of cottage cheese and yogurt are typically opaque.

Riboflavin deficiency results in dry cracked skin, especially around the mouth and nose. Eyes can also become sensitive to light. There is no known toxicity.

B3/Niacin

Niacin is another enzyme-producing B vitamin that assists the release of energy from cells. In addition, niacin helps control glucose levels in blood. It is also necessary for healthy nervous and digestive systems.

Niacin is found in high-protein foods such as fish, meat, poultry, peanuts, and in whole grains. When corn became a staple food of the poor throughout Europe, South America, and the southern United States, the niacin-deficiency disease pellagra became widespread. Symptoms include dermatitis, skin lesions, swollen tongue, mental confusion, aggression, and dementia.

The best source of niacin is the amino acid tryptophan, found in much of the animal protein you eat. Half of this amino acid is converted to niacin in the body. Vegans, who do not eat animal protein, run the risk of niacin deficiency.

B5/Pantothenic Acid

This vitamin, found in every food and made by intestinal bacteria, is important in the creation of enzymes that enable the conversion of fat and carbohydrates into energy. It is also important in hormone and red blood cell formation.

There is no recommended amount because it is so readily available in food. The best source for B5 is organ meat, but it is also plentiful in salmon, whole grains, eggs, beans, and milk. Frozen meat that has been defrosted, however, loses half of its pantothenic acid.

Deficiency has only been witnessed in lab studies and results in fatigue, mood swings, nausea, and cramps.

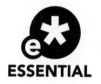

ESSENTIAL

Some endurance athletes claim pantothenic acid helps them train harder. Extra B5 is taken to better release energy from fats and carbs and to incur less lactic acid buildup. To date extensive research into these claims has not been conducted, however.

B6/Pyridoxine

This vitamin builds more than sixty enzymes, working for your immune and nervous systems and helping form red blood cells. It turns the protein you eat into proteins your body needs and helps convert carbohydrates into energy.

B6 is best found in high-quality protein foods such as chicken and fish. It occurs in dairy products, but not in large amounts, so again, vegetarians are frequently deficient. Deficiency symptoms include getting sick frequently because the immune system is weakened. Anemia, a low red blood cell count, is also common with B6 deficiency.

Some medications cause excretion of B6, including drugs for high blood pressure, asthma, arthritis, and birth control, as does alcohol. Toxicity is possible with large doses, more than 2,000 milligrams per day. B6 toxicity causes neurological damage. Symptoms can include tingling or numbness, and difficulty walking.

B9/Folic Acid

This vitamin is essential for strong bodies. It aids in protein metabolism, helps new red blood cell formation, and has been shown to prevent spine and brain birth defects and lower the risk of heart disease.

Beans are a good source of folic acid, as are spinach, asparagus, and chicken and beef liver. As with all water-soluble vitamins, folic acid is easily lost in cooking. Deficiencies cause anemia, nausea, sore tongue, headache, and weakness. Because B vitamins work together synergistically, if you're low in one you are usually low in them all.

Deficiency in folic acid can also be a sign of cancer. Cancer cells use up folic acid to fuel their cell division. Toxicity from folic acid is not a concern, as excess is excreted. Too much folic acid, however, can mask a rare type of anemia caused by a deficiency of B12.

FACT

Anemia is the most common blood disorder, classified as a deficiency of red blood cells or hemoglobin. It can be caused by loss of blood, destruction of red blood cells, or insufficient red blood cells. Symptoms include weakness, fatigue, lack of concentration, and in extreme cases, shortness of breath and heart failure.

B12/Colabamin

Found only in animal foods, B12 is crucial to maintaining healthy red blood cells, immune systems, and the development of genetic material. It helps the nervous system by strengthening the fatty layer of nerve cells.

Your body absorbs only about half of the B12 you ingest, therefore intake should be double what you need. Because it is found in animal foods, vegetarians may need supplements, as may the elderly. As people age, their bodies have difficulty absorbing B12, and the difficulty increases the older you get. Additionally, potassium supplements interfere with B12 absorption.

A condition known as pernicious anemia is caused by B12 deficiency. Other deficiency symptoms include pins and needles in hands and feet, numbness, depression, memory loss, and dementia.

Biotin, Choline, and Inositol

You do not need to consume these vitamins because they are made in adequate amounts by the bacteria in your intestines, but they are worth mentioning as they work closely with the other B vitamins, converting your food into energy. Biotin, in particular, helps you utilize fats and proteins. Choline and inositol work together in the formation of neurotransmitters, crucial for brain function, cell membranes, and to move fats out of your liver. Toxicity is unknown and deficiency is rare.

Vitamin C

This is arguably the king of all vitamins. Also known as ascorbic acid, vitamin C plays an important role in more than 300 functions in the body. It is the body's main antioxidant; it protects the immune system, helps build collagen for connective tissues, and heals wounds. Vitamin C is vital in the absorption of iron and calcium. It helps maintain blood vessels, bones, teeth, and the formation of brain hormones.

Vitamin C is associated with citrus fruit, which contains a lot of it, but vitamin C is also found in leafy greens, especially watercress, as well as kiwi fruit, peppers, potatoes, broccoli, strawberries, and tomatoes. Vitamin C requirements are increased by smoking, stress, allergies, birth control pills, antibiotics, and fever.

Deficiency results in scurvy, a disease whose symptoms include spots on legs, sore and bleeding gums, tooth loss, wounds that reopen, and eventually death. British sailors were given a daily ration of lime to prevent scurvy (that's where the nickname "limey" originated). Because such deficiencies are easily treatable with vitamin C, fatalities today are rare.

The Main Minerals

Minerals are not as easily destroyed by overcooking or improper handling as vitamins. Minerals are absorbed through your intestines and transported throughout the body by blood or proteins. These elements can be stored in various forms, so toxicity is a more serious concern. In fact, megadosing of minerals can be quite dangerous. Scientists are still learning about minerals, especially the trace minerals. Supplements are rarely needed, with the exception of iron, which is a very common deficiency.

Science has subdivided minerals into those you need more than 100 milligrams per day of, and those you need less than 100 milligrams a day of, known as trace minerals.

Calcium

This is the most abundant mineral in the body. You store 98 percent of it in your bones, 1 percent in your teeth, and the last 1 percent circulates around in your blood. It is extremely common for people to be deficient in calcium. Women are prone to deficiency, typically getting only about half of what they need from their regular diet.

Calcium is a crucial element in the normal formation of teeth and bones. With healthy amounts of calcium, human bone growth occurs naturally until middle age, at which time bone loss begins. Calcium deficiency limits growth throughout the early years, making adult bones thin and brittle. The effect can be slowed when calcium intake is increased.

Calcium also helps muscles contract. It is necessary for the production of enzymes and hormones involved in digestion and the conversion of nutrients into energy. It works with vitamin D to regulate blood calcium levels, and it helps blood clot.

Milk is the best source of calcium, but not the only one. Broccoli, kale, spinach, beans, and nuts are all excellent sources. Many foods, including cereal, orange juice, and bread, are fortified with calcium.

Calcium absorption can also be inhibited by certain drugs, including cortisone and other steroids, cholesterol-lowering drugs, thyroid drugs, antacids, alcohol, and tobacco.

Phosphorus

This mineral is found in all food, and the average diet provides plenty. Phosphorus works together with calcium to strengthen your bones and teeth. Like calcium, phosphorus circulates in the bloodstream and goes where it's needed, releasing energy from fat, protein, and carbohydrates. It also contributes to genetic material.

Like calcium, phosphorus is available in milk, as well as meat, poultry, fish eggs, beans, and whole grains. Phosphoric acid is also used in the production of soda pop. There are no good plant sources for phosphorus.

Magnesium

Magnesium is part of the pigment chlorophyll, found in green plants, including spinach and other green leafy vegetables. It can also be found in nuts, beans, and milk.

This mineral is in every tissue, and is necessary in the creation of energy-converting enzymes. It is also utilized in the formation of bones and teeth. Magnesium is used in the prevention of heart rhythm problems and high blood pressure. It is also thought to help prevent migraines and premenstrual syndrome (PMS).

Potassium, Sodium, and Chloride: The Electrolytes

Collectively, potassium, sodium, and chloride are referred to as the electrolytes. These electrically charged minerals dissolve in body fluid. They carry nutrients in and out of the cells, help send messages along the nerves, and control blood pressure. They are found throughout the body, dissolved in water. When you excrete liquids, your electrolytes need to be replaced.

Potassium is found in all living cells. A well-balanced diet contains lots of potassium derived from several sources, but certain foods are particularly high in potassium, including potatoes, legumes, prunes, and avocados. You are likely to get plenty of sodium and chloride because they are found in table salt—in fact, you probably get too much. They are not found just in the shaker, but in prepared foods, too.

Sports drinks are great for fluid and electrolyte recovery after prolonged activity. The liquid is absorbed quickly, and these drinks contain a good balance of nutrients. But they can be expensive. Make your own by blending ½ cup orange juice, 1 quart water, 1 teaspoon salt, and 1 tablespoon honey. Mix well and chill.

Potassium is found within the cells. Sodium and chloride remain outside the cells, in fluid. Sodium and chloride intake should never be higher than that of potassium. A healthy intake that keeps fluids in balance is considered to be five parts potassium to one part sodium and chloride. If that ratio changes, high blood pressure results. High blood pressure can lead to heart disease, kidney disease, and stroke. Potassium exists in almost every food, but because most people consume too much salt, they need to supplement with potassium to stay in balance.

Chloride is also part of hydrochloric acid, the acid in your stomach that aids digestion and kills bad bacteria. It's not a mineral you need to worry about, though. Because you probably get plenty of salt in your diet, you are getting enough chloride.

Sodium and Your Health

What is commonly called table salt is sodium chloride (NaCl). It is a combination of the two minerals sodium and chloride, in a 40:60 ratio. You need both minerals, but only in very small quantities. They occur naturally in most foods, but you get the majority of your sodium from manufactured food products. Canned soups and vegetables, condiments, baked goods, chips, and other snack foods are loaded with added salt. It is used in preserving, stabilizing, and flavoring.

As an electrolyte, sodium is essential to keep your body fluids in balance, regulate your blood pressure, spark nerve impulses, relax muscles, and digest proteins and carbohydrates.

How Much Salt?

There is no recommended amount of sodium, because people are in no danger of deficiency. Modern Americans consume 4,000 to 6,000 milligrams of salt every day. The recommended limit is 2,400 milligrams (just under 1 teaspoon), but your body only needs about 400 milligrams a day (less than ¼ teaspoon).

Excessive sodium intake can be problematic. Eating too much sodium on occasion is not uncommon, but most of it is excreted in sweat and urine, with the help of your kidneys. You may have experienced a bloated feeling after a particularly salty meal. You most certainly experienced the thirst that follows. Thirst is your body's attempt to regulate fluid balance by sending water to the cells, commonly referred to as water retention. The craving is the body's way of telling you to drink up.

Sodium and High Blood Pressure

When the kidneys don't work properly to rid the body of excess sodium, a swelling in your feet and legs occurs, known as edema. Excessive sodium intake is a contributing factor to osteoporosis, as well as high blood pressure, also known as hypertension.

As blood flows through your arteries, pressure is created against the arterial wall. If sodium is not eliminated, it accumulates in the blood. Water is added to compensate for the imbalance and blood volume increases, leading to high blood pressure. High blood pressure, or hypertension, is a result of too much pressure being placed on the arterial wall.

Hypertension is considered a risk factor in coronary artery disease, kidney disease, and stroke. Although not a direct result of sodium intake, elevated sodium levels in combination with other risk factors, including age, heredity, obesity, smoking, alcohol consumption, and limited physical activity, can lead to health problems.

Decreasing Your Sodium Intake

If you are concerned about your sodium intake, you have several options. Simply cutting back slowly is probably the best course of action. Unless you have serious hypertension and your doctor has instructed you to quit cold turkey, cut back slowly and let your taste buds become accustomed to the flavor of the foods themselves, not the salt.

Check the labels of the foods you regularly buy, then choose lower sodium replacements. Salt substitutes are another option, unless you have a sensitivity to potassium. Most substitutes replace at least a portion of sodium chloride with potassium chloride.

Keep track of your daily salt intake. Nutrition fact panels on packaged and canned foods have made it easy to determine how much salt you're eating. Total up the daily value percentage of sodium in the foods you consume each day, and try to keep it at or below the 2,400 milligrams recommended limit. Check out the recipes later in this chapter for some delicious salt substitutes.

QUESTION

How can I easily reduce my salt intake?
First of all, taste your food before you salt it. You may find it tastes fine as it is! Also, do not salt your food as you cook it. Instead, use only the salt on the table. You'll add less overall, and you'll notice it more. Another trick for reducing salt intake is to abandon the salt shaker in favor of the old-fashioned salt cellar. This is a small covered container with a tiny spoon. You have more control over how much salt you use, and you'll use less.

Herbal and Other Seasoning Mixtures

Using herbs is a delicious way to season dishes and cut the amount of salt needed for flavor, too. Although fresh herbs need to be used immediately, dried herb mixtures can be prepared in advance and stored in an airtight container. The easiest way to dry fresh herbs is to put the baking sheet in an oven at 200°F–225°F for 1 hour. Blends made from whole seeds or leaves usually need to be coarsely ground in a spice grinder or small food processor prior to using.

Barbecue Blend

4 tablespoons dried basil
4 tablespoons dried rubbed sage
4 tablespoons dried thyme
4 teaspoons cracked black pepper
4 teaspoons dried savory
1 teaspoon dried lemon peel

Cajun Blend

2 tablespoons paprika
1½ tablespoons garlic powder
1 tablespoon onion powder
½ tablespoon black pepper
2 teaspoons cayenne pepper
2 teaspoons dried oregano
2 teaspoons dried thyme

Caribbean Blend

1 tablespoon curry powder
1 tablespoon ground cumin
1 tablespoon ground allspice
1 tablespoon ground ginger
1 teaspoon ground cayenne pepper

Country Blend

5 teaspoons dried thyme
4 teaspoons dried basil
4 teaspoons dried chervil
4 teaspoons dried tarragon

Fish and Seafood Herbs

5 teaspoons dried basil
5 teaspoons crushed fennel seed
4 teaspoons dried parsley
1 teaspoon dried lemon peel

French Blend

1 tablespoon crushed dried tarragon
1 tablespoon crushed dried chervil
1 tablespoon onion powder

Herbes de Provence

4 teaspoons dried oregano
2 teaspoons dried basil
2 teaspoons dried sweet marjoram
2 teaspoons dried thyme
1 teaspoon dried mint
1 teaspoon dried rosemary
1 teaspoon dried sage leaves
1 teaspoon fennel seed
1 teaspoon dried lavender (optional)

Italian Blend

1 tablespoon crushed dried basil
1 tablespoon crushed dried thyme
1 tablespoon crushed dried oregano
2 tablespoons garlic powder

Mediterranean Blend

1 tablespoon dried sun-dried tomatoes
1 tablespoon dried basil
1 teaspoon dried oregano
1 teaspoon dried thyme
1 tablespoon garlic powder

TIP: If you don't have a food processor, you can freeze the sun-dried tomatoes so they will be easier to crush; however, that adds moisture to the herb blend, so it can't be stored.

Middle Eastern Blend

1 tablespoon ground coriander
1 tablespoon ground cumin
1 tablespoon turmeric
1 teaspoon ground cinnamon
1 teaspoon crushed dried mint

Old Bay Seasoning

1 tablespoon celery seed
1 tablespoon whole black peppercorns
6 bay leaves
½ teaspoon whole cardamom
½ teaspoon mustard seed
4 whole cloves
1 teaspoon sweet Hungarian paprika
¼ teaspoon mace

Pacific Rim

1 tablespoon Chinese five-spice powder
1 tablespoon paprika
1 tablespoon ground ginger
1 teaspoon black pepper

Sonoran Blend

1 tablespoon ground chili powder
1 tablespoon black pepper
1 tablespoon crushed dried oregano
1 tablespoon crushed dried thyme
1 tablespoon crushed dried coriander
1 tablespoon garlic powder

Stuffing Blend

6 tablespoons dried rubbed sage
3 tablespoons dried sweet marjoram
2 tablespoons dried parsley
4 teaspoons dried celery flakes

Texas Seasoning

3 tablespoons dried cilantro
2 tablespoons dried oregano
4 teaspoons dried thyme
2 tablespoons pure good-quality chili powder
2 tablespoons freshly ground black pepper
2 tablespoons ground cumin
2 small crushed dried chili peppers
1 teaspoon garlic powder

CHAPTER 9

Food Labels

Our government has played a role in food labeling for about twenty years. It's interesting to learn about the foods you are eating; however, the labels you see on packaged and canned foods can be a bit confusing. Some of the information provided on food labels is helpful, but some is couched in convoluted terminology or marketing hype. This chapter will make you aware of what exactly you need to focus on and what you can skip over with confidence.

Food Label History

Food labels have been mandatory in the United States since the 1990s, but they have been in the making since the 1860s. What began as an agricultural research and development project quickly morphed into a food safety organization. After the Civil War, as interstate commerce picked up, a need arose for standardized weights, measures, and manufacturing practices.

FACT

After the Civil War, each state had its own food regulations. It was common for food companies to produce different versions of the same product, in varying degrees of quality, to comply with different state laws.

By the 1870s, concern about the quality of traded goods prompted the Pure Food and Drug Movement. Activists urged lawmakers to make food adulteration a crime. At the time, chemical preservatives went uncontrolled, milk was unpasteurized, and ice provided the only form of refrigeration. Cottonseed oil was routinely sold as lard, and glucose syrup made from wheat and corn was used as a cheaper form of sugar. Unbeknownst to the consumer, medical "tonics" routinely contained opium, morphine, cocaine, and heroin. In 1903, volunteer "poison squads" ate foods tainted with chemical preservatives to demonstrate their effect on human health.

How to Read Nutrition Labels

You'll want to look at several key areas of a food label. The first and most obvious is the front of the package. There you will find graphics designed to appeal to a specific consumer. For instance, bright colors and cute or goofy characters are aimed at kids. Also on the front you'll see the product's claims: "Tastes Great" and "New and Improved" are the tame, long-standing ones. It's the health claims consumers need to pay attention to. "Heart-Healthy," "Whole Grain," and "Less Sugar" are claims designed to draw the attention of health conscious, but not necessarily nutritionally savvy, shoppers.

Somewhere on the package you'll find a list of ingredients and the nutrition facts panel. Pay attention to these.

The Nutrition Facts Panel

Nutrients listed on the facts panel were chosen because of their importance in relation to modern health issues. New listings appear as health concerns change. For example, the listing for trans fat is a relatively recent addition. Placement on the label is an indication of importance, too. For instance, sodium is not listed with the other minerals and micronutrients, but up high, next to cholesterol, because many people need to monitor their sodium intake.

A label is placed on every food package, either vertically or horizontally. Sometimes you have to search a bit, as folds in the packaging can hide it. Sometimes, too, the label is on the box, but not on individually packaged contents inside.

FACT

Labels are not required on most food served for immediate consumption, such as that sold in bakeries or delis, or served on airplanes or in hospitals. But if a restaurant makes specific health and nutrient claims, then labels (typically on a separate sheet) must be provided upon request.

Serving Size

The top of the panel lists the serving information. The serving size is the quantity of the product on which the facts are based. The facts are not based on the entire package. If you do not read the serving size, the rest of the information is useless.

Serving sizes are often shocking. For instance, a regular four-inch bagel may constitute two or more servings; a serving of cookies may be just one cookie. Do not be misled by a low calorie count. Check the serving size before you get excited.

Don't forget to take the food's preparation, if any, into consideration. Serving size may be before or after water or other ingredients are added. This information will also be printed clearly in the serving size area of the label.

Servings per Container

This little bit of information is useful if you tend to eat an entire package of food in one sitting. It will tell you how many servings the package contains. All it takes is some easy math to figure out just how many servings, and thus how many calories and grams of fat, were in that bag of chips you just consumed.

Percent Daily Value

Daily values (also known as daily reference values, or DRVs) show you how much of the daily recommended nutrients are in the product. The figure is given as a percent of a designated amount of nutrients required for a 2,000-calorie-per-day diet. The recommendations are high and considered the most that would be healthful for adults.

The percentage listed on the label is based on a recommendation of total daily nutrients. These daily nutrient percentages are as follows:

- Fat should constitute 30 percent of calories.
- Saturated fat should constitute 10 percent of calories.
- Carbohydrates should constitute 60 percent of calories.
- Protein should constitute 10 percent of calories.
- Fiber is based on 13 grams daily.

If you are on a special diet, these percentages may not apply.

RDI

The term "recommended daily allowance" is being replaced by "reference daily intake" (RDI). During World War II, investigations into diet and nutrition prompted the establishment of a recommended daily allowance. Information gained in those studies was put to use in the armed forces, the civilian population, and in overseas relief efforts. The RDIs are the equivalent to the RDAs, and are used to determine the daily reference value percentages.

Calories

Calories measure energy. They are determined by burning a weighed portion of food, and measuring the heat it produces. Different nutrients contain different amounts of calories. Carbohydrates and proteins each contain four calories per gram, fat has nine calories per gram, and alcohol has seven calories per gram.

In prepared foods with numerous ingredients and varying portion size, the calorie designation is useful and welcome information. However, be careful not to limit your label reading to the calorie section. Low calories often mean low nutrition. Knowledge of calories is only a small part of your healthy eating arsenal.

Fat, Carbohydrates, and Protein

The nutrition facts panel gives a general listing for fat, followed by sub-listings for saturated fat and trans fat, two forms of fatty acids that should be as close to zero as possible in healthy diets. (See Chapter 7 for more information about fat.) You'll also see listings for cholesterol and sodium, two nutrients that should be limited as well.

Carbohydrates are listed as a total figure, as well as being separated into fiber and sugar. Fiber is a carbohydrate that, while indigestible, is still vital for good health. Fiber helps keep digestion flowing, and maintains normal cholesterol and blood sugar levels. There is no daily value percentage for sugar because it is not a recommended nutrient.

Protein is generally not a nutrient most Americans need to be concerned with. We get plenty of it, so listing its daily value percentage is not required unless the product is marketed as a high-protein food, as in baby food or meal replacements. Often the grams per serving is all that is listed.

Vitamins and Minerals

The only required listings in this section are vitamin A, vitamin C, calcium, and iron. The average diet is often deficient in these micronutrients. Products may choose to add more information about vitamins and minerals if the product contains significant quantities.

What are micro- and macronutrients?
Vitamins and minerals are considered micronutrients because only small quantities are necessary for good health. (Micro comes from the Greek *mikros*, meaning small.) Carbohydrates, protein, fat, and water are considered macronutrients, as you require much larger quantities of them. (Macro comes from the Greek *makros*, meaning long.)

Recommended Daily Limits

On larger packages, just below the vitamins and minerals, you may find a list of the daily limits of nutrients. These numbers, listed as quantities in grams, are based on a 2,000- and 2,500-calorie diet. This is a nice reminder of overall dietary needs. For a 2,000-calorie diet, the daily limits are as follows:

- Total fat should not exceed 65 grams.
- Total saturated fat should not exceed 20 grams.
- Total cholesterol should not exceed 300 milligrams.
- Total sodium should not exceed 2,400 milligrams.

Nutritional Claims

It's hard to find a label that doesn't make some sort of claim, hoping you'll add the product to your shopping cart. But when you see the words "free" or "light" on the label, can you believe them? According to the FDA, you can. Manufacturers are required to provide scientific evidence before they are allowed to make claims on labels. Twelve terms are strictly regulated: free, low, reduced, less, lean, extra lean, light/lite, more, fewer, high, good source, and healthy.

Free

A label claiming to be calorie-free must contain less than five calories per serving. Sodium-free, sugar-free, and fat-free foods must contain less than .5 grams per serving. "Cholesterol free" means the product has less than 2 milligrams of cholesterol per serving, and 2 grams or less saturated fat per serving.

Low

"Low calorie" means the product has forty calories or less per serving. "Low fat" products must have 3 grams of fat or less per serving. "Low cholesterol" means less than 20 milligrams per serving and 2 grams or less of saturated fat per serving. "Low sodium" must have 140 milligrams or less per serving. "Very low sodium" means 35 milligrams or less.

Reduced

A product labeled "reduced" must have at least 25 percent less of the nutrient than the food it is referencing. For example, reduced-fat salad dressing must have 25 percent less fat than regular salad dressing.

Less

A product labeled "less" must have 25 percent less of a nutrient than the food it is referencing. For example, chicken broth labeled as having less sodium must have 25 percent less sodium than regular chicken broth.

Lean and Extra-Lean

"Lean" foods must have 10 grams or less of total fat, 4.5 grams or less of saturated fat, and 95 milligrams or less of cholesterol per serving or per 100 grams. "Extra-lean" foods can have no more than 5 grams total fat, 2 grams saturated fat, and 95 milligrams cholesterol.

Light or Lite

Products labeled "light" must have one-third fewer calories per serving than the food it is referencing, or 50 percent less fat than the reference food. If the product gets over 50 percent of its calories from fat, it must reduce the fat by another 50 percent to carry the "light" descriptor. Light sodium means the product has 50 percent less sodium per serving.

More

Products labeled "more" must contain at least 10 percent of the daily reference value of the nutrient in question. Synonyms for the word "more" on packages include "fortified," "enriched," "added," "extra," and "plus."

Fewer

Requirements for claims of "fewer" are the same as those for "reduced." The product must contain at least 25 percent less of the nutrient than the referenced product.

High

Products with "high" on the label must contain 20 percent or more of the daily reference value of vitamins, minerals, fiber, or protein.

Good Source

If a product claims to be a "good source" of something, it must have 10–19 percent of the daily value of that vitamin, mineral, fiber, or protein.

Healthy

Perhaps the most crucial word of all, the "healthy" claim, has several criteria. The food must provide at least 10 percent of the daily value of vitamins, minerals, fiber, or protein. If it is a meal product (meant to serve as an entire meal, such as a frozen dinner), it must contain 10 percent of the daily value of at least two of those nutrients. Sodium may not exceed 360 milligrams, or 480 milligrams for a meal product. The product must also follow the criteria for low fat, low saturated fat, and low cholesterol.

Health Claims

Claims regarding specific health issues are strictly regulated by the FDA. The words "may" and "might" must appear as a part of such claims.

These claims are powerful. If a product meets the criteria, its label can state that the product may prevent cancer, or brain damage, or heart disease. These claims are exciting, but it's important to note that these products do nothing in terms of prevention unless combined with a healthy lifestyle.

Many products link themselves to prevention of a certain disease. Claims regarding osteoporosis must contain 200 milligrams, or 20 percent of the daily value of calcium, and must be low in fat. Low-fat, low-saturated-fat, and low-cholesterol foods, and extra-lean meats may claim to help prevent cancer and coronary heart disease. These claims can also be made for high-fiber foods that meet the "low-fat" criterion and the "good source" criterion for fiber and vitamin A or vitamin C. Soy protein products for the prevention of cancer must meet the low-fat criterion and carry at least 6.25 grams of soy protein per serving.

Other Claims

"Percent fat-free" products must meet the low-fat or fat-free criterion. The percentage used must reflect the amount of fat in 100 grams of the product.

Some products try to imply health. Stating a product is made with a nutritious product, such as soy or bran, is not allowed unless the product can meet the "good source" criterion.

The term "fresh" can be used if the product is raw or unprocessed. This means it has never been frozen or heated, and it contains no preservatives. This is used in products such as fresh mozzarella cheese, sold in brine, and dated for freshness. Fresh-frozen products are frozen while still fresh in the orchards or on fishing boats. Some blanched and low-irradiated products may be called fresh as well.

ALERT

Claims that imply health through inclusion of certain ingredients are particularly problematic when new health and nutrition reports are in the news. To be sure what you're buying is all it claims to be, check the FDA website, *www.fda.gov*, for up-to-the-minute information.

You may also find one or more stamps on various food products. Here are just a few you might run into:

- **Whole Grain Stamp:** Helps you easily identify whole grains in the supermarket. You can visit *http://wholegrainscouncil.org* to view a list of approved whole grains.
- **American Heart Association Stamp:** Found on products that coincide with a heart-healthy diet.

- **MyPyramid.gov Stamp:** Provides percentages of daily grains, fruits, and vegetables per serving.
- **Smart Choices Program Guiding Food Choices:** This is often shown on the package as Smart Choices Made Easy. It helps guide more nutritious food choices in nineteen different food categories. It also includes front-of-pack calorie information.
- **Fruits & Veggies More Matters:** This brand logo may appear on all fruits and vegetables that have only water added and comply with other criteria set by the Centers for Disease Control and Prevention (CDC). Criteria can be found at: *www.fruitsandveggiesmatter.gov /health_professionals/program_guidelines.html.*
- **3 Every Day Milk, Cheese, and Yogurt:** The National Dairy Council provides a logo for guiding healthy dairy product options. Visit this website to learn more: *www.nationaldairycouncil.org/recipes/Pages /RecipeLanding.aspx.*

The Ingredients List

Ingredients are listed on products according to weight, from most to least. The food's main ingredient will be listed first. This is important to know, especially when looking at sweetened foods. If the food contains only one ingredient, such as a bag of dried beans, no ingredient list is required.

Ingredient lists are vital to people with allergies. It is estimated that 8 percent of children in the United States have food allergies. Of these, 90 percent are caused by one of eight foods: milk, eggs, peanuts, wheat, soy, fish, shellfish, and tree nuts. These eight foods must be listed on an ingredients list if they are used in the product. Color additives, too, must be acknowledged in the ingredients list by name, as well as soy-based flavor enhancers and milk derivatives called caseinates, commonly used in nondairy products. Beverages that claim to contain a specific juice must list the percentage of that juice.

Familiarizing yourself with the ingredients list, the nutrition facts panel, and the labeling laws is an eye-opening experience. Take a look at the foods you have in your cupboard right now and see how they rate. You may be surprised.

CHAPTER 10

Nutrition for Women

Knowing how your nutritional needs can change throughout your life span can help you gracefully adjust to ensure you feel your best. All too often, women put themselves and their needs on the back burner, focusing instead on family, friends, and loved ones and losing all sense of priority. Although it's important for us to take care of others, our ability to do so may decline if we don't care for ourselves first. Certain medical conditions that are specifically related to women require the need for some nutritional background.

Pregnancy

Good nutrition should always be a priority, but when you're having a baby it becomes even more important. At this period in your life it is vital to stick to good health habits. Ensuring you receive all of the nutrients your body needs will help to promote a safe pregnancy and a healthy environment for your baby.

Pregnancy and Weight Gain

Proper weight gain is vital to a healthy baby and a safe pregnancy. A baby's birth weight is directly related to the weight you gain throughout your pregnancy. A woman who is at a healthy weight at the onset of pregnancy should expect to gain anywhere from twenty-five to thirty-five pounds during the course of the pregnancy. Women who are underweight are advised to gain twenty-eight to forty pounds, and women who are overweight are advised to gain fifteen to twenty-five pounds. If you are expecting twins, your doctor may advise a weight gain of thirty-five to forty-five pounds.

Not only is gaining a healthy amount of weight important, but the rate at which you gain is also significant. Woman should expect about a two- to four-pound weight gain during the first trimester and about a one-pound gain per week for the remainder of the pregnancy.

▼ **Where Does the Weight You Gain Go?**

Baby	7–8 pounds
Placenta	1–2 pounds
Amniotic fluid	2 pounds
Breasts	1 pound
Uterus	2 pounds
Increased blood volume	3 pounds
Body fat	5 or more pounds
Increased muscle tissue and fluid	4–7 pounds
Total	minimum 25 pounds

Pregnancy and Calorie Needs

Calorie needs increase during pregnancy to help support a woman's maternal body changes and the baby's proper growth and development.

The RDI for energy intake during pregnancy is an additional 300 calories per day for the second and third trimester, in addition to maintenance needs. For example, if you require 2,000 calories per day to maintain your weight, you will need about 2,300 calories during pregnancy.

ALERT

Dieting or skipping meals during pregnancy can have serious effects on the development of the baby. It takes more than 85,000 calories over the course of a nine-month pregnancy, in addition to the calories the mother needs for her own energy needs, to produce a healthy, well-developed baby.

All the calories you consume during pregnancy should be healthy calories that contain plenty of protein, complex carbohydrates, fiber, vitamins, and minerals. Complex carbohydrates such as fruit, whole-grain starches, cereal, pasta, rice, potatoes, corn, and legumes should be the main source of energy.

Protein Power

Protein needs increase when you are pregnant to help develop the body cells of the growing baby. Other changes that are taking place in your body during pregnancy, such as the building of the placenta, also require protein. You need an extra 10 grams of protein above your extra daily calories or about 70 grams of protein daily, compared with 60 grams for women who are not pregnant. Ten grams of protein is equivalent to an ounce-and-a-half serving of lean meat, about 10 ounces of fat-free milk, or 1½ ounces of tuna canned in water.

Most women do not have a problem meeting their protein requirements. Consuming plenty of lean meats, fish, tuna, eggs, and legumes, as well as increasing your dairy servings, will ensure you meet your protein needs. If you are a vegetarian, consume a variety of legumes, grain products, eggs, low-fat or fat-free dairy products, vegetables, fruits, and soy foods to ensure proper protein intake.

Adjusting Your Eating Plan

Getting the extra calories your body needs for pregnancy just takes a small adjustment in a healthy eating plan. Adjust your eating plan using the following guidelines for the minimum number of servings in each food group:

- Bread, cereal, rice, and pasta group: 6–7 (or more) servings daily
- Vegetable and fruit groups: 5 or more servings daily
- Milk, yogurt, and cheese group: 2–3 servings daily
- Meat, poultry, fish, dried beans, eggs, and nut group: 5–7 ounces daily
- Unsaturated fats: 3 servings daily

Also be aware of increased fluid needs. Water is an important nutrient and is essential for the nourishment that passes through the placenta to the baby. Drink at least 8 to 12 cups daily and more if you are thirsty.

ALERT

Eating raw foods can increase your risk for bacterial infection. Avoid anything raw, including sushi and other raw seafood, undercooked meat or poultry, beef tartar, raw or unpasteurized milk, soft-cooked or poached eggs, and raw eggs (possibly found in eggnog).

Vitamin and Mineral Needs

Vitamin and mineral needs also increase with pregnancy. Unlike calorie needs, your increased need for vitamins and minerals is immediate. Certain ones are especially important, such as folate, calcium, and iron.

Folate

Folate is especially important for women during the first three months of pregnancy. The body uses folate to manufacture new cells and genetic material. During pregnancy, folate helps develop the neural tube, which becomes the baby's spine. Because most women do not know that they are pregnant immediately, and because the neural tube and brain begin to form so soon after conception, getting enough folate on a regular basis is important if you are of childbearing age. Taking enough folate can help to greatly reduce the risk of neural tube birth defects such as spina bifida and birth defects of the brain (anencephaly). The National Academy of Sciences recommends women of childbearing age get 400 micrograms (mcg) of folate each day, especially one month prior to conception.

FACT

National surveys show the average folic acid intake by women of childbearing age is about 230 micrograms daily. Folic acid intake should be kept below 1,000 micrograms per day to avoid excessive intake.

Most women get folic acid daily through fortified products and other foods. To get more folic acid in their diets, women anticipating pregnancy should eat more citrus fruits and juices, leafy dark-green vegetables, legumes, and fortified breakfast cereals. To ensure adequate intake, woman can take a multivitamin that contains folic acid in addition to eating a healthy diet.

Not all vitamin supplements contain folic acid, so check the label to make sure about the amount. Also, not all multivitamin supplements are optimal before or during pregnancy. Pregnant women and those anticipating pregnancy should consult their doctors for advice about taking folic acid or any other vitamin or mineral supplement.

Vitamin A

Vitamin A is important for promoting the growth and health of cells and tissues throughout your body and the baby's. A healthy diet should provide enough vitamin A during pregnancy so there is no need for a supplement.

New research has shown that consuming too much vitamin A, in excess of 10,000 IU daily, may increase the risk of birth defects. This is twice the RDA. Eating foods such as fruits and vegetables that are high in beta-carotene is not a problem because beta-carotene does not convert to vitamin A when blood levels of vitamin A are normal.

Other Vitamins

With your increase in calorie intake, your increased need for most of the B vitamins will be met through your dietary intake. Vitamin B12 is found in animal foods such as milk, eggs, meat, and cheese. Women who are vegetarian and don't consume any type of animal foods need to make sure they consume a reliable source of vitamin B12, such as fortified breakfast cereals and/or a B12 supplement. If you don't feel you are meeting your B12 needs, talk to your doctor before taking supplements.

Vitamin C needs increase slightly but can be met easily by consuming an extra glass of orange juice, an orange, or another citrus fruit. Vitamin C is important because it helps the body absorb iron from plant sources, and iron needs almost double during pregnancy.

Vitamin D is essential because it helps the body to absorb extra needed calcium. A glass of vitamin-D-fortified milk will take care of your extra needs. If you're a vegetarian who does not consume dairy products, your doctor may prescribe a supplement. Make sure your doctor knows your eating habits.

Pumping Up Calcium and Iron

Two minerals that deserve special attention are calcium and iron. If you don't consume enough of either of these minerals throughout your pregnancy, the baby will actually use the calcium in your bones and the iron in your blood.

ALERT

The estimated calcium needs for pregnant girls under eighteen is 1,300 milligrams per day. For pregnant adult women aged nineteen to fifty, the recommended intake is 1,000 milligrams per day. There is also an Upper Tolerable Limit for pregnant women set at 2,500 milligrams per day.

Although it is important to get calcium throughout your life, it is especially important during pregnancy. Calcium helps ensure that your bone mass is preserved while the baby's skeleton develops normally. Consuming plenty of calcium before, during, and after pregnancy can also help reduce your risk for osteoporosis later in life. Good sources of calcium include dairy products and some green leafy vegetables. If you are vegetarian or lactose intolerant and do not eat dairy products, consume plenty of other good calcium sources, such as calcium-fortified orange juice or calcium-fortified soy milk, along with special lactose-reduced products.

An increase in the blood volume of a pregnant woman greatly increases her iron needs. A woman's need for iron increases to 30 milligrams per day. Several foods supply iron, including meat, poultry, fish, legumes, and whole-grain and enriched grain products. Iron needs during pregnancy can be more difficult to meet because iron isn't always absorbed well, and many women have low iron stores before they get pregnant. Most prenatal vitamins contain iron, and your doctor may also prescribe an iron supplement. Keep in mind, though, that supplements are just to help out; you still need to eat a diet rich in iron. Iron from plant sources is not as easily absorbed as that from animal sources. Eating a good source of vitamin C, such as citrus fruits or juices, broccoli, tomatoes, or kiwi, with meals will help the body absorb the iron in the foods you eat. The absorption of iron from supplements is best when the stomach is empty or when taken with juice containing vitamin C.

Menstruation

A woman's menstrual cycle involves a delicate interaction of hormones and physiological responses. The menstrual cycle is the body's way of preparing itself every month for a possible pregnancy. As women of childbearing age go through menstruation, overall nutrition is an important issue.

Boosting Iron

During a woman's years of menstruation, iron needs are a special nutritional concern. On average, women lose about ¼ cup of blood at each menstrual cycle; women with a heavy flow may even lose more. Because iron travels through the blood, some of it is lost with the loss of blood.

Women of childbearing age have an RDI of 15 milligrams per day for iron, which doubles during pregnancy. Women over the age of fifty-one have a lower RDI of 10 milligrams per day because most of them have reached menopause and are no longer losing blood (and therefore iron) each month.

It is common for women of childbearing age to become iron deficient. A deficiency of iron can cause fatigue and weakness. Deficiency can also lead to anemia. The combination of iron lost through the menstrual cycle, a low dietary intake of iron, frequent dieting, and a low intake of vitamin C all contribute to the problem of iron deficiency.

It is helpful not only to eat iron-rich foods, but also to take a multivitamin supplement that contains iron. Many supplements contain iron and are designed for women with that in mind. Check your supplement to make sure it contains iron.

ALERT

If you take both an iron and calcium supplement, take them separately, at different times of the day. They will both be better absorbed if taken on their own.

Iron can be found in both animal products and plant sources, but the iron from meat is better absorbed than that in plant foods. Certain nutrients, such as vitamin C, can help enhance the absorption of iron from plant sources. For example, you can increase the amount of iron the body can use from iron-containing plant foods by drinking a glass of orange juice. Good sources of iron include meat, poultry, fish, fortified cereal, enriched rice, and legumes.

Premenstrual Syndrome (PMS)

Premenstrual syndrome, or PMS, afflicts many women. This condition can have several symptoms and varying degrees of severity from woman to woman. The exact cause of PMS is not completely understood, though experts believe that hormones such as progesterone, estrogen, and testosterone are probably involved. A change in the level of serotonin in the brain is also believed to be related to the occurrence of PMS. For most women the symptoms of PMS seem to appear after ovulation, or about fourteen days into the cycle, and disappear two weeks later, as the menstrual period starts. PMS is closely tied with mood swings, bloating from water retention, tender breasts, headaches, temporary weight gain, and food cravings.

Avoiding certain foods can help. Some of the following foods may exacerbate your symptoms: caffeine, simple sugars, salt or sodium, fats, and alcohol.

Even though food cravings and other symptoms may be a predictable part of PMS, some things can be done to help relieve some symptoms. Foods that may help to relieve some symptoms include complex carbohydrates and high-calcium foods. Stick to a diet that includes plenty of fresh fruits and vegetables, whole-grain products, nonfat dairy products, lean fish, and poultry; also drink plenty of water. Be sure to exercise regularly, too. Exercise can help release tension and anxiety, and it promotes the release of endorphins, which naturally sedate you.

You may have heard that certain supplements and vitamins help to relieve the effects of PMS. At one time vitamin B6 was believed to ease PMS symptoms, but solid evidence was never found, and taking too much B6 was harming many women. To get the possible benefits of B6, consume foods rich in the vitamin, including fish, chicken, soy foods, broccoli, bananas, cantaloupe, and spinach. Until more is known, your best bet for relieving PMS symptoms is to follow some general guidelines. Eat an overall healthy diet, lead an active lifestyle, get plenty of sleep, and consult your doctor if needed.

Menopause

Menopause is the natural part of a women's life cycle when the menstrual period stops. A natural life event, it marks the end of the childbearing years. It is sometimes called "the change of life" and is a unique and personal experience for every woman.

In technical terms, menopause occurs when the ovaries run out of eggs and decrease the production of the sex hormones estrogen, progesterone, and androgen. Women experience menopause at various ages, but most go through it around age fifty. It is considered an early menopause at any age younger than forty to forty-five.

QUESTION

Are there other factors that will affect the age at which I hit menopause?
Genetics is definitely a key factor, so knowing your family history may give you a clue. Also, cigarette smoking can cause menopause to occur two years earlier for women who smoke than for nonsmoking women.

Changes and signs of menopause include the following:

- Hot flashes (sudden warm feeling, sometimes with blushing)
- Night sweats (hot flashes that occur usually at night and can often disrupt sleep)
- Fatigue (probably from disrupted sleep patterns)
- Mood swings
- Early morning awakening
- Vaginal dryness
- Fluctuations in sexual desire or response
- Difficulty sleeping

Many of the symptoms as well as health problems of menopause are due to the decreasing levels of estrogen. Treatment with estrogen (estrogen replacement therapy, or ERT) or with estrogen and progestin (hormone replacement therapy, HRT) has been used to help relieve some of these symptoms and supposedly decrease the risk for certain health problems such as heart disease and stroke. Approximately 25 percent or 8 million American menopausal women currently take ERT or HRT. Taking ERT or HRT may help to reduce symptoms of menopause, but it is now uncertain whether the risks outweigh the benefits. Doubt exists as to whether ERT and HRT really do decrease the risks of certain health problems, and there are contraindications in taking HRT for women who have a history of cancer. Taking HRT and ERT is an extremely complicated issue with many pros and cons. Every woman should assess her own personal needs and discuss her options with her doctor. If you're taking these replacements, it is important to have regular medical checkups.

ESSENTIAL

An ongoing study being done by the National Institutes of Health called the Women's Health Initiative (WHI) is studying the effects of both ERT and HRT on women. Due to their recent findings, they have asked the women in the study to stop using HRT. They concluded that HRT does not prevent heart disease and is not beneficial overall. The jury is still out on the benefits of taking estrogen (ERT) alone. Scientists at WHI are continuing to study and analyze the use of ERT and HRT. You can find updated information at *www.nih.gov* and *www.whi.org*.

Current research is now examining soy foods as an alternative treatment for the symptoms of menopause. These soy foods contain phytoestrogen (also called isoflavones), a plant hormone similar to estrogen. Research is still in its beginning stages, and much more needs to be established before any conclusions can be made.

Health Issues and Menopause

At least two major health problems can develop in women in the years after menopause: heart disease and osteoporosis. A decrease in hormone production is most likely the cause of these conditions at this stage in life. The years following menopause can be healthy years, depending on how you take care of yourself. Not all women will develop heart disease or osteoporosis after menopause. Many lifestyle factors can affect your heart and your bones that have nothing to do with estrogen levels. The key to helping prevent heart disease and osteoporosis is lifestyle change, with nutrition and physical activity as major components.

Weight Gain in Menopause

Perimenopause, which leads to menopause, marks the beginning of the end of the menstrual cycle. In this stage, which lasts from five to ten years, estrogen levels begin to decline, ovulation becomes less regular, and weight gain tends to become a problem. Some women who have struggled with just a few extra pounds often find themselves struggling harder against weight gain during perimenopause. Even women who have generally been in a healthy weight range for many years suddenly find themselves having to work a lot harder to stay there.

Some experts believe the reason for weight problems is the fluctuation in hormone levels, whereas others suggest it is an age-related decline in muscle mass that ultimately decreases metabolism. Dieting isn't the only answer, however. The key is lifestyle change and exercise combined. Experts feel that if you have not been exercising throughout your life, perimenopause is the time when you should really begin. At this stage in your life you need to develop more muscle mass through exercise to achieve a higher, fat-burning metabolic rate that can help you lose extra pounds and stay at a healthy weight.

Heart Disease

Many serious health concerns affect women, but none is more serious than heart disease, the nation's leading killer. The American Heart Association says that "nearly one million people die from heart disease yearly." Heart disease is often thought of as a man's disease, but that is a misconception. Even though breast cancer is most often quoted as the number one cause of death in women, nearly six times as many women die from heart disease. In 1996, women's deaths from heart disease outpaced men's by 505,930 to 453,297. The facts tell it all: one in nine women over age forty-five and one in three women over sixty-five have coronary heart disease. Approximately half of all women will eventually develop some form of heart disease.

Until menopause, estrogen reduces the likelihood of plaque buildup in the arteries and acts as protection from heart disease. After menopause, a woman's risk steadily increases for developing coronary artery disease, or CAD, a condition in which the veins and arteries leading to the heart become narrowed and/or blocked by plaque. Heart attack and stroke are caused by CAD, in most cases.

ESSENTIAL

Estrogen helps to raise HDL cholesterol (good cholesterol), which helps remove LDL cholesterol (bad cholesterol) that contributes to the accumulation of fat deposits called plaque along artery walls.

Women need to concentrate on making heart-healthy choices throughout life, but especially in the years after menopause. It is important to eat a diet that is low in total fat, saturated fat, and cholesterol; eat plenty of grain products, vegetables, and fruits; stay physically active; keep a healthy weight; control stress levels; go easy on sodium; and consult with a doctor about hormone replacement therapy.

Osteoporosis

Osteoporosis is a brittle-bone disease that increases the risk of bone fractures later in life. Osteoporosis afflicts more than 8 million women and 2 million men. More than 80 percent of osteoporosis sufferers are women; osteoporosis affects half of all women over the age of fifty and almost 90 percent of those over the age of seventy-five. Five to 20 percent of women die each year due to osteoporosis-related complications.

Your Risks for Osteoporosis

Menopause is the single greatest risk for osteoporosis. Others include gender, age, family history, hormone deficiencies, low calcium intake, excessive alcohol and caffeine consumption, and cigarette smoking. Estrogen helps prevent bone loss and works together with calcium and other hormones and minerals to help build bones. When women hit menopause and are not making as much estrogen, their risk for osteoporosis increases. Try to prevent osteoporosis in your younger years instead of treating it after menopause. The stronger and healthier your bones are when you enter menopause, the more bone mass you will have to sustain you as you age.

Bone loss varies from woman to woman. Osteoporosis prevention should include a balanced diet rich in calcium and vitamin D. From childhood through early adulthood, adequate calcium helps build bone mass; in the late postmenopausal years, eating plenty of calcium-rich foods and taking a calcium supplement can help slow bone loss. Experts also recommend participating in weight-bearing exercises such as walking, and avoiding smoking and excessive caffeine intake.

FACT

The RDI for women after menopause, not taking hormone replacement therapy, is 1,500 milligrams of calcium daily; for women who do take HRT, the RDI is 1,200 milligrams of calcium.

How to Handle Osteoporosis

Osteoporosis has no actual cure, but some treatments and preventive measures can help to slow or reverse bone loss and help prevent fractures. Try some of these tips:

- **Increase your calcium intake to 1,000–1,500 milligrams per day.** As you age, your body absorbs and uses calcium less efficiently. Foods high in calcium include dairy foods, green leafy vegetables, shellfish, sardines with bones, oysters, brazil nuts, fortified tofu, and almonds. Many foods available today such as orange juice, breads, breakfast cereals, and soy milk are fortified with calcium.
- **Weight-bearing exercise that actually puts weight on your bones—** weight resistance training, walking, jogging, aerobic dance, or tennis— can help promote bone health.
- **Consult your doctor about whether taking hormone replacement therapy (HRT) is right for you.** Combined with exercise and adequate calcium intake, HRT may help prevent bone loss, but the benefits may not outweigh the risks.
- **Reduce your caffeine intake** (about 40 milligrams extra dietary calcium is needed to offset the amount of calcium lost from one cup of coffee).
- **Drink alcohol in moderation.** People who drink heavily have less bone mass and lose bone more rapidly.
- **Stop smoking.** People who smoke have a greater risk of fracture. Also, women who smoke have lower estrogen levels. Estrogen helps protect you from osteoporosis.

It is advised that women be evaluated for osteoporosis if they fracture easily, are sixty-five or older, or are menopausal with other risk factors. If left completely untreated, a postmenopausal woman can lose 10 to 40 percent of bone mass between the ages of fifty and sixty.

Aging

As you age your caloric needs decrease because you have more body fat and less lean body mass. It is more important than ever to balance nutritional intake, because you require the same nutrient needs but fewer calories. Use the following tips from the Young at Heart Tips for Older Adults. Visit *http://win.niddk.nih.gov/publications/young_heart.htm* to read the complete guide.

- **Do not skip meals.**
- **Make sure to eat high-fiber foods** such as vegetables, fruits, whole-grain breads and cereals, and beans at each meal to help balance energy levels, maintain heart health, and promote bowel regularity.
- **Choose lean beef, turkey breast, fish, or chicken.**
- **Vitamin D is essential.** Eat fortified low-fat/fat-free milk, yogurt, or cheese every day. If you are lactose intolerant or choose not to consume milk products, try reduced-lactose milk products, soy-based beverages, or tofu. You may also supplement with calcium and vitamin D.
- **Choose foods fortified with vitamin B12.** Many adults over the age of fifty have difficulty absorbing adequate amounts of B12.
- **Limit your consumption of high-fat and high-sugar snacks** such as cake, candy, chips, and soda.
- **Drink plenty of water,** even if you feel less thirsty.

Life changes in many ways as we age, including our living situations. Several local programs such as Meals on Wheels make it easier for senior citizens to get the nutritious meals they need. Call the Eldercare Locator at 1–800–677–1116 for information about the program nearest you. A great way to stay social and stretch your budget is to grocery shop with someone else. You can plan recipes together, split the cost of ingredients, prepare extra for several meals that you can store in the freezer, and have fun.

CHAPTER 11

Nutrition for Men

This chapter includes information specific to men in terms of nutritional needs, certain medical conditions, and what to eat as you get older. It's important to realize that it's never too late to make lifestyle changes, no matter what habits you may have developed since childhood. Trying new foods or incorporating more physical activity into your daily life can have cumulative healthy benefits. Being a role model for friends and family is a goal anyone can achieve.

Cholesterol

Cholesterol is a waxy, fatlike substance found in tissue and in the blood. Our bodies manufacture about 80 percent of our cholesterol supply, and we get the rest by eating certain foods, especially saturated fats. Cholesterol that is found in food is called dietary cholesterol; the type found in your bloodstream is referred to as blood or serum cholesterol. Many factors affect blood cholesterol. The cholesterol that circulates in your body comes from both the cholesterol your body produces and from the foods you eat. Even though you often see cholesterol listed with dietary fat, cholesterol is not the same as fat.

FACT

When triggered by sunlight, cholesterol in your skin has the ability to convert to vitamin D, which is an essential vitamin necessary for building bone.

Cholesterol differs from fat in that it possesses a different type of structure and performs separate functions in the body. Cholesterol also differs from fat in that it is not broken down in the body and therefore does not provide energy and calories. Eating too much fat can cause you to gain weight, whereas cholesterol cannot.

Cholesterol is essential for maintaining healthy cell function. The body requires it to insulate nerves, create cell membranes, and produce certain hormones such as estrogen and testosterone. It is part of every body cell and is also a component of bile, which helps the body to digest and absorb needed fat. In moderation, cholesterol is essential to many bodily functions. However, your body makes plenty of cholesterol, and most dietary cholesterol you consume is considered to be excess.

Computing Your Cholesterol

It is important to have your blood cholesterol checked regularly because symptoms of high cholesterol are not always obvious. The American Heart Association recommends that all adults aged twenty or older have a fasting lipid profile (total cholesterol, LDL cholesterol, HDL cholesterol, and triglyceride) once every five years.

Cholesterol is measured through blood analysis and is best tested when the person fasts for at least twelve hours prior to drawing blood. The sample is analyzed for total cholesterol and, if the need exists, for LDLs and HDLs. Cholesterol is measured in milligrams per deciliter (mg/dL).

Triglycerides

Triglycerides don't get as much attention as cholesterol, but they are also linked to heart disease. If you have several risk factors for heart disease, your doctor will probably check your triglyceride levels along with your cholesterol. Triglycerides are the main form of fat in foods and in the blood. Your triglyceride level will fall into one of these categories:

- **Normal:** less than 150 mg/dL
- **Borderline to high:** 150–199 mg/dL
- **High:** 200–499 mg/dL
- **Very high:** greater than 500 mg/dL

Because of their roles in metabolism, triglyceride levels are inversely related to HDL-cholesterol levels. When a person has a high triglyceride level, the HDL-cholesterol levels are usually low.

Total Cholesterol Levels

It is important to ask your doctor for a total lipoprotein profile so you are aware of not only your total cholesterol but of each component of your cholesterol. You may have a total cholesterol level that is desirable, but that doesn't mean your HDL and LDL levels are in line. Your total cholesterol level will fall into one of three categories:

- **Desirable:** less than 200 mg/dL
- **Borderline high risk:** 200–239 mg/dL
- **High risk:** 240 mg/dL and over

If you fall in the desirable range, your risk for heart attack is relatively low. However, it is still smart to get plenty of physical activity and to follow a healthy diet low in cholesterol and saturated fat, and to maintain a healthy weight.

If you fall within the borderline high-risk range, you have at least twice the risk of a heart attack compared with someone who is in the desirable range. If you are in this range, your HDL is less than 40 mg/dL, and you don't have other risk factors for heart disease, you should have your total cholesterol and HDL rechecked in one to two years. You should also lower your intake of foods high in saturated fat and cholesterol to help reduce your cholesterol level to below 200. Your doctor may order another blood test to measure your LDL cholesterol. Even if your total cholesterol puts you in the borderline high-risk range, you may not be at high risk for a heart attack. Some people, such as women before menopause, and young, active men with no other risk factors, can have high HDL cholesterol and desirable LDL levels, so it is best to ask your doctor to interpret your results. Everyone's case is different.

FACT

The American Heart Association now encourages Americans to think of their blood cholesterol as a vital sign, similar to blood pressure, for measuring heart health.

If your total cholesterol level is 240 or more, you are definitely at high risk. Your risk of heart attack and, indirectly, of stroke are greater. If you fall in this category, you should ask your doctor for advice. About 20 percent of the U.S. population has what are considered high blood cholesterol levels.

The bottom line is that the less LDL you have, and the more HDL you have, the lower your risk for heart disease. When it comes to trying to lower your LDL, your food choices are key.

Follow your physician's advice after you have had your cholesterol tested.

If you have a cholesterol reading over 240 mg/dL or you have risk factors such as heart disease along with cholesterol readings over 200 mg/dL, your doctor will probably prescribe a cholesterol-lowering medication in combination with a healthy low-fat diet and exercise. Several different types of these medications are on the market today, and your doctor may even prescribe more than one. Your doctor should periodically test your blood cholesterol levels to check on your progress. As with any type of medication that your doctor prescribes, it is essential to follow the recommended dosage and schedule requirements to experience results.

Diabetes

In the United States, approximately 18 million people have diabetes, 12 million of them men. Diabetes is a disease that prevents the body from producing or properly using insulin. Insulin is a hormone that the body needs to convert sugar, starches, and other food into energy for daily life. In healthy people, insulin helps regulate blood sugar levels. People with diabetes have trouble controlling blood sugar.

FACT

Today, the incidence of Type 2 diabetes is nearing epidemic proportions. This is in large part due to the increased number of older Americans, the increased rate of obesity, and the increase in sedentary lifestyles of Americans.

There are two major types of diabetes. In Type 1 diabetes, the body does not produce any insulin. This type most often occurs in children and young adults, but not always. People with Type 1 diabetes must take a daily injection of insulin to survive. Type 1 diabetes accounts for 5 to 10 percent of diabetes cases.

In Type 2 diabetes, the body does not make enough insulin or use it properly. This is the most common form of the disease. Type 2 diabetes accounts for 90 to 95 percent of all people with diabetes. Obesity is a major risk factor for developing Type 2 diabetes.

Complications

Many complications are associated with diabetes, and most are strongly related to high blood sugar levels. In fact, with its complications, diabetes is the seventh leading cause of death in the United States. It is estimated that each year at least 190,000 people die as a result of diabetes and its complications. Keeping your blood sugar levels in your target range is your best defense against the complications of diabetes.

Complications can include the following:

- Blindness
- Heart disease and stroke
- Kidney disease
- Nerve disease and amputations
- Gum disease
- Impotence
- Skin disorders

To lower your risk of these complications, get regular checkups, be aware of warning signs, keep blood sugar levels close to normal, control your weight, eat a healthy, well-balanced diet, get regular exercise, do not smoke, and check your feet every day for minor cuts or blisters and show suspicious ones to your health-care practitioner.

Symptoms

In some instances, diabetes can go undiagnosed because some of the symptoms seem so mild and/or harmless. Recent studies indicate that early detection and treatment is the key to decreasing the complications of diabetes later on.

Diabetes symptoms may include:

- Frequent urination
- Increased fatigue
- Excessive thirst
- Irritability
- Extreme hunger
- Blurry vision
- Unusual weight loss

If you have one or more of these symptoms, you should see your doctor immediately.

Managing Diabetes with Diet

Managing diabetes with diet means eating well-balanced, healthy meals. Along with nutrition, other lifestyle modifications such as exercise, a healthy weight, and medications (insulin or oral diabetes pills) are essential to diabetes control. Controlling diabetes means keeping blood sugar levels as close to normal (nondiabetic level) as possible.

In the past, strict diets for diabetics were used, but recently they have become more flexible. Following a "diabetic diet" is really no different from that of a typical healthy diet for a person without diabetes. Diabetics should limit fat, sodium, and sugar intake. They should also eat plenty of fruits, vegetables, whole grains, and fat-free or low-fat dairy products.

ESSENTIAL

Work closely with a registered dietitian to design a meal plan that is right for you—one that fits into your lifestyle and includes foods you enjoy. A diabetic meal plan acts as a guide to show you how much and what types of foods you should choose for meals and snacks.

Fiber is an important part of a healthy diet and can also be helpful in controlling blood sugar levels. The soluble type of fiber from legumes, oats, fruits, and some vegetables may help slow the rate at which sugar is absorbed into the bloodstream. This can keep blood sugar levels from rising rapidly.

The main goal is to choose a plan that will help you to control your blood sugar levels. It is important that diabetics learn how to self-manage their condition as well as their diet.

A Type 1 diabetic's plan will require coordinating food intake with the action of the insulin he or she is using. A Type 2 diabetic's plan will involve restricting calories for weight loss, gaining knowledge about better food choices, and eating small meals or snacks every couple of hours throughout the day, rather than the usual three big meals. Reducing your weight by just ten to twenty pounds has been shown to lower high blood sugar levels. Eating small portions more frequently throughout the day can help to keep insulin and blood sugar levels more stable.

With treatment, blood sugar levels may go down to normal again. But this does not mean a diabetic is cured. Instead, a blood sugar level in the target range shows that the treatment plan is working and that the diabetes is being managed correctly.

Exercise

Exercise, along with good nutrition and medication, is also important for diabetes control. Increasing activity helps the body transport glucose to your cells. It also helps lower blood sugar levels and reduces the risks for heart disease and obesity. Exercise usually lowers blood sugar, which enables your body to use its food supply better. Also, exercise may help insulin work better. Your health-care provider can assist you in deciding what kinds of exercise and how much exercise are best suited to your needs. If your blood sugar control is poor, do not exercise. Get medical advice first.

Weight Control

Often, men who have been involved in sports or physical activities early in life run into weight gain later when their activity levels change. It is important to always focus on basic nutrition, and to include a high volume of vegetables and fruits in your diet. Busy work schedules may cause you to skip lunch or go too long without eating between meals. This is extremely common among men, and can make the goal of long-term weight loss more challenging. Set up your office to support you and your health by keeping nutrient-dense foods on hand. If you're on the road, bring along a travel bag or cooler filled with healthy foods so you won't skip meals. Keep in mind when you are balancing your nutrition, you are a better role model for your whole family.

Aging

Over time, the accumulated wear and tear on your body could promote illness or injury. Therefore, it's important to do proper, routine maintenance checks periodically to assess your health—just as you would do for your car. The best ways to prevent illness or injury are to complete recommended screening tests suggested by your doctor, don't smoke, eat a healthy diet, stay physically active, and maintain a healthy weight.

According to the U.S. Preventive Services Task Force, screening tests for men should check for obesity, high cholesterol, high blood pressure, colorectal cancer, diabetes, depression, sexually transmitted infections, HIV, and abdominal aortic aneurysm. Following recommendations from the dietary guidelines will help ensure you take preventative measures.

CHAPTER 12

Nutrition for Babies and Kids

Eating habits and lifelong attitudes toward food are often formed at an early age. Parents can take advantage of the first few years of life to guide and educate children about the most important foods for growth, strength, mental clarity, and overall health. The good thing is that kids are extremely receptive to new ideas. The tips in this chapter will help support you in shaping your child's future.

When and What Toddlers Should Eat

You can give a child solid foods as early as six months of age, but it is not until the second year of life that regular patterns of eating take hold. Year two is also a time when problems may arise. As children begin sitting at the table and eating meals with the family, eating patterns begin to change. Social cues are learned and behaviors are enforced. The more you know in the early stages, the fewer problems you will have later on with your child's nutrition and food-related behavior.

As children grow, it is the parents' job to help them become independent eaters, so that eventually they will take responsibility for their own nutrition. The earlier the quest for independent eating begins, the more successful it will be. Here are some easy things you can do to get your children off on the right foot:

- **Be a good example.** Eat a wide variety of healthy foods in sight of your child. Avoid the foods you want your child to avoid.
- **Set a schedule.** Well-planned meals and snacks at regular times keep kids' blood sugar levels balanced and prevent hunger that is typically accompanied by whining, crankiness, and lack of cooperation.
- **Teach your kids that food is fuel.** Like gas in the minivan, it gives them energy to get through the day. Do not use food as a reward, a weapon, a punishment, or a substitute for love.

First Whole Foods

Several theories exist regarding what is the best progression to solid foods. The fact is, so long as you take the foods one at a time, and are mindful of balancing the child's diet, the order of foods isn't important. However, as your child begins to feed himself, new considerations must be taken into account, especially the dangers of choking.

Hot dogs and grapes lead the list of foods kids choke on, followed by nuts, raw carrots, popcorn, and hard candies. The size and shape of these foods are just right for lodging in the trachea and blocking airflow through it.

Most of these foods are not recommended for young children anyway, so by following a sensible diet, your child is already better off. Although few children are allergic to hot dogs, they are not a good source of protein. Yes, they are easy to eat, mild, and most kids gobble them up. But they are loaded with saturated fat, sodium, and sugar. Children are better off eating boiled chicken or turkey.

Trying New Foods

Continue to introduce new foods to your child, but do not force them. This is a period when food plays an important role, both good and bad, in your child's life. It can make her feel more grown up, or give her control over you.

When you introduce something new to a toddler, it's best to place no more than one or two tablespoons of it on the plate. Do not announce it or let them know it is new. Do not watch in anticipation, or warn them they may not like it. Just sit down and eat it too. If they don't like it, and many will not, let it go for this meal, but try it again another night. Sometimes it takes a dozen tries before a child will try something new. The key is to not make a fuss about it. If this refusal to eat gets attention, the behavior will continue, even if the attention is negative.

FACT

Distaste and fear of food contamination is common in toddlers. It could be a natural survival mechanism, meant to prevent recently mobile kids from eating everything in sight. Foods that look, smell, and taste weird to them are often immediately rejected.

New foods or textures mixed into familiar foods are frequently detected because a child's palate is more sensitive than an adult's. Not only will the food be rejected, but the parent will lose trust.

Foods that the child believes resemble something gross (such as noodles that look like worms) may be rejected. Often, anything touching the "worms," or merely on the same plate, will also be rejected by association. Forcing the issue in cases like this can make matters worse, leading to retching and vomiting. Letting matters get to this point has the potential for a long-term negative association with that food, and the battle is lost.

ESSENTIAL

Food jags are common among kids of this age. A "jag" is when they insist on eating only one food for breakfast, lunch, and dinner. A jag can last for a week or two, but there is no need to worry about malnutrition. If it goes on longer, help break the cycle by including kids in grocery shopping and cooking.

Kids who don't eat are a worry to their parents. The fear of malnutrition makes parents constantly offer their kids food. But the loss of appetite is usually the parents' fault. Often kids are given too much milk and juice. Toddlers should not drink more than sixteen ounces of milk a day, and no more than four ounces of 100-percent juice. Parents should also limit snacking, especially sweet snacks. If kids fill up on these things throughout the day, they will have little appetite when family mealtime rolls around.

Portion size is another area of concern. Kids do not need adult-size portions, but food labels are based on adult portion sizes. As previously discussed, you should relate your portion size to the palm of your hand. The same is true for a toddler. Look at his hand and use it to judge portion size. If you want to be more precise, a toddler should be getting about 1,300 calories a day, or 40 calories per inch of height. This is about one-quarter of the food an adult needs.

To help ensure those 1,300 calories mean something nutritionally, use the following guidelines, based on the dietary recommendations in Chapter 2:

▼ **Toddler Dietary Guidelines**

Food	Toddler Servings
Whole Grains	6
Vegetables	3
Fruit	2
Milk	2
Meat/Protein	2

When and What Older Kids Should Eat

Breakfast, lunch, midmorning and afternoon snacks, and dinner should fulfill a child's nutritional needs if you follow the dietary guidelines. But skipping meals, excessive snacking, and lack of exercise can throw a kid's diet out of balance.

Breakfast is the most important meal for school-age kids, as well as for adults. If kids are hungry midmorning, they will have poor concentration and difficulty with mental functioning. Breakfast does not need to be limited to traditional breakfast foods. It's worth taking time to find nutritious foods kids will eat willingly, rather than fighting through the meal or letting them skip it.

A brown bag lunch is preferable to one from a school cafeteria. School lunches are typically packed with fat, sodium, and sugar, and are overcooked to the point of diminished nutrient content. They usually don't taste very good, and they can do some damage to the positive food attitudes you have been trying to build. Select what goes into the brown bag with care. By lunchtime children will be hungry and will need healthy energy, not sugar-packed juice drinks and junk food.

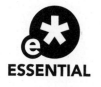

ESSENTIAL

Snacks are a useful way to stave off hunger and to ensure all daily nutrients are being consumed. But this only works if the food is nutritious, so keep healthy snacks in the house. Veggie sticks, cheesy popcorn, and cereal are excellent choices. High-fiber, low-sugar snacks provide stamina, so kids can get through their homework without nodding off from a sugar crash.

By dinnertime, if your kids have been eating nutritiously in appropriate quantities all day, they will probably be ready to clean their plates. One way to ensure they'll eat what's put in front of them is to make sure they get a daily dose of vigorous exercise before dinner to round out the day's healthy activities.

Food and School

When kids enter school they are confronted with new experiences and challenges, which include food and eating. Here, among their peers, pressure to fit in begins, often in the lunch room. Even if you pack their lunches, kids will inevitably trade, bargain, and auction off sweet snack cakes and candy. Arm your school-age children with nutritional smarts.

They should know what constitutes a healthy diet before they lay eyes on the lunch lady. Teach them which foods will make them fat, tired, or sick, and which foods will make them strong and healthy. Before they enter school, get them used to skim milk, vegetables, fruits, and whole grains. Limit the extras, such as ice cream and candy. Sweets should be fruit, and desserts should be reserved for special occasions.

The food you send to school with your children should be as healthy as the food they eat at home. Avoid prepackaged lunches. They are typically loaded with sodium, fat, and sugar. The lunch line may not be much better. Even if the school offers "healthy" choices, there is no guarantee that's what the kids will pick.

Picky Eaters

After age five, parents no longer need to worry about the adequate calorie intake of their children. The problem now lies in limiting caloric intake. That is why it is particularly important to monitor the quality of the calories kids eat and the way they conduct themselves at the table.

FACT

Sixty percent of American toddlers eat pastry every day. Ten percent of American babies four to six months old consume sweets, including soda pop. Baby food companies do not put sugar in their fruits and vegetables, but they do sell baby dessert. Remember, a child's sweet tooth is easily placated by fruit.

If your child is a difficult eater, you don't need to bend over backward to please her. Part of growing up is learning to eat politely and show respect.

As a parent, you should not tolerate persnickety behavior. But in keeping with the idea of a calm, stress-free family table, try not to let the pickiness instigate conflict. Here are a few tips:

- Be upbeat and calmly explain that they are expected to taste everything. If they do not like it, that's fine, but there will be no more food offered that evening.
- Don't force them to clean the plate. Don't badger them to eat something. Food taste is a very personal thing. What is perfectly acceptable to one may be distasteful to another. Arguing over it is pointless. You can ignore it or simply state, "Too bad. Maybe someday you'll like it."
- Do not make multiple meals. You are not a short-order cook. If they are hungry, they will eat.

Encouraging Experimentation

One of the greatest things about food is the immense variety of it. Kids who are offered a wide variety of foods during weaning are less likely to be persnickety older children. By age five they are old enough to try new cuisines, both when eating out and in the comfort of home.

One way to interest kids in new foods is to interest them in the place it came from. Get a map and pick a country. Or pick a place they're interested in—maybe one they're studying in school—and look for related foods.

If your kid is fascinated with ancient Egypt, find out what Egyptian cuisine is all about. If your kid likes music, learn about the food eaten in the music capitals: Nashville (barbecue), New Orleans (gumbo), or Mozart's Austria (schnitzle and sacher torte). If it's sports they love, learn about the native cuisine of favorite players, or the famous food of the team's hometown. Every subject can somehow be related to food in a fun and interesting way.

Childhood Obesity

The percentage of overweight children, aged six to seventeen years, has doubled in the United States since 1968. In 1994 one in five children were considered obese; today one in three children in the United States are over-weight. Studies also show that almost 70 percent of overweight kids aged ten to thirteen will be overweight or obese as adults.

ALERT

An increasing number of teenagers are also overweight, and, if no in-tervention is made, approximately 80 percent of them will stay over-weight or become obese as adults.

Children and teens may experience psychological and emotional fall-out from being overweight as youngsters. They may struggle with self-esteem and be teased by other children. Overweight children are also put at risk for health problems. Studies show that overweight children tend to have higher levels of blood sugar, blood pressure, and blood fats.

Children can become overweight for a variety of reasons. The most common are genetic factors, lack of physical activity, unhealthy eating pat-terns, or a combination. In rare cases, a medical problem can cause a child to become overweight.

Assessing whether a child is overweight can be difficult because chil-dren grow in erratic spurts. If you feel your child or teen may be overweight, consult your family physician. Your doctor may use growth charts to deter-mine if there is a problem.

Handling an Overweight Child

Children and teens should never be placed on a calorie-restricted diet to lose weight unless they are under the strict supervision of a doctor for medical reasons. Limiting what children or teens eat can be harmful to their health and can interfere with proper growth and development. It can also be psychologically stressful for a child. Helping children to adopt healthy eating and exercise habits is more important than encouraging them to sim-ply lose weight. Behavior modification strategies have shown considerable success in effecting long-term weight loss. The best programs incorporate plenty of physical activity and healthy eating, including slowing the rate of eating, limiting the time and place of eating, and teaching problem-solving through exercises. The most effective treatments also involve parents.

ALERT

Although limiting fat intake may help prevent excess weight gain in children, it is not a good idea to restrict fat intake in children who are younger than two.

To help your child achieve a healthy weight, try the following techniques:

- **Seek the advice of a health-care professional,** such as a registered dietitian or doctor. Keep in mind that adult approaches to weight loss are not fit for children.
- **Give your children support, acceptance, and encouragement, no matter what their weight, and talk to them about their feelings.** This will help them carry a positive self-image, making weight loss more achievable.
- **Starting in early childhood,** teach children proper nutrition, how to select healthy low-fat snacks, and the importance of physical activity. Monitor the time they spend watching television or sitting at a computer.
- **Provide good nutrition at family meals, and make exercise a family affair.** Serve low-fat meals to the entire family, keep nutritious snacks in the house, and plan family activities. This will help the child feel part of the family instead of isolated (and the whole family will benefit).
- **Beware of using food as a reward,** as a substitute for affection, or as a compensation for a disappointment. Choose other avenues as rewards.
- **Make sure your child's portions are a child's as opposed to an adult's size.** Use smaller plates for children so you or the child is not tempted to fill up a large plate.
- **Explain to children how to recognize when their bodies tell them that they are hungry or full.**

- **Stock your kitchen with low-fat and low-calorie snack foods,** so they are available when the child is hungry. Avoid bringing high-fat, high-calorie foods into the house.
- **Instead of heavy snacking, make meals the primary source of calories.**
- **Do not encourage children to continue eating or clean their plates when they are truly no longer hungry.**
- **Avoid labeling foods as "good" or "bad."** Instead, help your child to learn how to fit all types of food into a healthy eating pattern, and teach them how to eat foods in moderation. Even if your child has a few pounds to lose, he or she can still eat foods such as sweets in moderation. What counts is the diet as a whole.
- **Make a family rule that eating is only allowed in the kitchen or dining room,** to keep kids from snacking on high-calorie foods while watching television. Children will most likely eat less with this rule in place.

Recipes

Avocado Mash

Avocado is a great first food. It's loaded with monosaturated fat (the good fat), folate, potassium, and fiber. Avocados do have more calories than other fruits and vegetables, so use in moderation.

INGREDIENTS | YIELDS 6 TABLESPOONS

1 ripe avocado

Can You Freeze an Avocado?

Avocados do not freeze well due to their consistency. You can use lemon juice on the avocado to help prevent browning; however, your baby is not ready for citrus until closer to one year old, so only cut the amount of avocado that you can use in that day. Or, make the family guacamole and pull some plain avocado out for your baby.

1. Slice avocado around the outside lengthwise. Twist both sides off the seed of the avocado. Scoop out flesh from one side of the avocado. Mash until desired consistency reached.

2. Wrap remaining avocado with the seed in it with plastic wrap and store in the refrigerator.

PER TABLESPOON Calories: 40 • Fat: 3.5 g • Carbohydrates: 2 g • Protein: 0.5 g • Sodium: 1.5 mg • Fiber: 2 g

Apple, Pumpkin, and Barley Cereal

Pumpkin purée adds a creamy texture to this combination.

INGREDIENTS | YIELDS 6 TABLESPOONS

2 tablespoons prepared iron-fortified barley cereal (with either breast milk or formula)

2 tablespoons apple purée

2 tablespoons pumpkin purée

Combine all ingredients.

PER TABLESPOON Calories: 20 • Fat: 0 g • Carbohydrates: 4 g • Protein: 0.5 g • Sodium: 0.5 mg • Fiber: 1 g

Organic Jarred Applesauce

Organic applesauce can be combined with cereal and breast milk or formula, mixed with a vegetable purée, or just served on its own. Most brands have a very smooth consistency that works well even for beginning eaters. If the texture is lumpy, you should purée it for baby.

Chicken, Banana, and Coconut

This is a great dish for grownups, too! Cook the adult portion in a separate pot so you can spice it up by adding red chili paste, diced onions, curry powder, and/or fresh cilantro. Serve over brown or Arborio rice.

INGREDIENTS | SERVES 2

6 cups water
1 boneless, skinless chicken breast
1 small banana or ½ large banana
1 teaspoon coconut milk

1. In a large pot bring 6 cups of water to a boil. Place the chicken breast in the pot and boil until done, approximately 10 minutes. Cut into small pieces and allow to cool.

2. Combine chicken, banana, and coconut milk in a food processor or blender until desired consistency is reached. Use broth from cooking the chicken, breast milk, or iron-fortified formula to reach an age-appropriate consistency. If consistency is too chunky, drain through a sieve and purée remaining liquid.

PER SERVING Calories: 113 • Fat: 1.5 g • Carbohydrates: 8.5 g • Protein: 18 g • Sodium: 0.5 mg • Fiber: 1 g

Homemade Applesauce

Make a stockpot full of this delicious sauce during the fall, and freeze in 1-cup containers.
It will stay good for up to six months in your freezer.

INGREDIENTS | SERVES 3

3 sweet apples
⅛ teaspoon cinnamon
Enough water to cover apples

Applesauce for Baking
You'll find recipes for baked goods in this book that use applesauce mixed with baking powder. Homemade applesauce is perfect for this. Mash the applesauce to a smooth consistency and then follow the baking recipe directions.

1. Peel apples and cut into chunks. In a large saucepan, combine apple chunks and cinnamon. Cover apples with water. Cook until apples are very tender and start to break apart.

2. Mash with a potato masher or the back of a spoon. Transfer to blender or food processor if a finer consistency is needed.

PER SERVING Calories: 50 • Fat: 0 g • Carbohydrates: 15 g • Protein: 0 g • Sodium: 0 mg • Fiber: 2 g

Peaches and Quinoa

Quinoa has been grown in South America for more than 6,000 years. The Incas revered quinoa as the "mother of all grains" due to its unique nutritional properties. It has a good amount of balanced protein and is high in fiber, phosphorous, magnesium, and iron.

INGREDIENTS | YIELDS 6 TABLESPOONS

2 ounces of peach purée
1 tablespoon cooked quinoa

1. Combine peach purée and cooked quinoa.

2. If necessary, use a food processor or blender until desired consistency reached.

PER TABLESPOON Calories: 12 • Fat: 0 g • Carbohydrates: 2 g • Protein: 0.5 g • Sodium: 0 mg • Fiber: 0.5 g

Apple and Sweet Potato Mini-Muffins

*Because these muffins aren't too sweet they're great as a take-along snack,
warmed and topped with butter or sweet potato spread.*

INGREDIENTS | YIELDS 42 MINI-MUFFINS

2 cups white whole-wheat flour
1½ teaspoons baking powder, divided
½ teaspoon salt
½ teaspoon cinnamon
½ cup applesauce
½ cup flaxseed meal
¼ cup canola oil
½ teaspoon vanilla
½ cup milk (dairy or soy)
1 cup frozen apple juice concentrate
1½ cups grated sweet potato
1 cup grated apple

1. Preheat oven to 350°F.

2. In a medium bowl, combine flour, 1 teaspoon baking powder, salt, and cinnamon.

3. In a large bowl, combine applesauce with ½ teaspoon baking powder.

4. Add flaxseed meal, oil, vanilla, milk, and apple juice concentrate. Stir to combine.

5. Slowly mix dry ingredients into wet.

6. Mix in sweet potato and apple.

7. Pour batter into a lightly oiled mini-muffin pan.

8. Bake for 25–30 minutes or until a toothpick inserted in the middle of a muffin comes out dry.

PER MUFFIN Calories: 52 • Fat: 2.3 g • Carbohydrates: 7 g • Protein: 1.5 g • Sodium: 33 mg • Fiber: 1.5 g

Oatmeal with Sautéed Plantains

Plantains are a Central American staple; they can be cooked in sweet or savory dishes.

INGREDIENTS | SERVES 4

1 yellow plantain (very ripe)
1 tablespoon brown sugar
1 teaspoon butter
½ cup water
½ cup apple juice
⅔ cup rolled oats
1 teaspoon ground cinnamon

Plantains Versus Bananas

Plantains are firmer and have a lower sugar content than bananas. Plantains need to be cooked, but bananas are mostly eaten raw. In tropical areas of the world, plantains are often a first food for babies. Plantains are a staple item in these areas and are consumed on a daily basis.

1. Peel and cut plantain into ½" pieces.

2. Put brown sugar in a plastic bag and place plantain pieces in bag, shaking the bag to coat them.

3. Heat butter in a small pan over medium heat; place plantains in pan and cook until the sugar begins to caramelize, about 2 minutes each side; remove from heat.

4. In a small saucepan, combine water and apple juice. Bring to a boil.

5. Once boiling, stir in rolled oats and cinnamon. Return to a boil.

6. Reduce heat to low and simmer to desired thickness, 3–5 minutes.

7. Top oat mixture with sautéed plantains and serve.

PER SERVING Calories: 167 • Fat: 3 g • Carbohydrates: 34 g • Protein: 4 g • Sodium: 14 mg • Fiber: 3 g

Couscous with Grated Zucchini and Carrots

Butter or oil added to this dish prevents the couscous from forming clumps or curds. Remember, your baby needs fat for healthy brain and eye development.

INGREDIENTS | SERVES 6

1 cup whole-wheat couscous

1 cup water

2 tablespoons butter or canola oil

1 teaspoon ground flaxseeds

½ cup zucchini, grated

½ cup carrot rounds

½ teaspoon garlic

1 teaspoon oil

1 cup canned white beans

How Do You Use Flaxseeds?

Purchase fresh flaxseeds. Store them in the refrigerator and grind them right before use. Get an inexpensive coffee grinder that you use specifically for this purpose. Grind in small batches and store in an airtight container in the fridge. Use these quickly once they have been ground.

1. Add couscous, water, and butter or canola oil in a microwaveable glass bowl. Cover and heat on high for 2–3 minutes. Remove from microwave and fluff with fork. Sprinkle ground flaxseeds on couscous and blend with fork.

2. Place carrot rounds and zucchini in a microwaveable bowl and steam until tender.

3. In a medium saucepan, sauté garlic in oil over medium heat until clear.

4. Add beans to cooked zucchini and carrots and heat through.

5. Combine couscous, beans, zucchini, and carrots.

PER SERVING Calories: 276 • Fat: 7.6 g • Carbohydrates: 42g • Protein: 12 g • Sodium: 17 mg • Fiber: 8 g

Creamy Cauliflower Soup

For added texture, remove one-third of the soup before puréeing.
After soup is puréed, return to pot and combine with reserved soup.

INGREDIENTS | SERVES 6

½ onion, chopped

1 tablespoon olive oil

3 medium potatoes, peeled and diced

1 medium head cauliflower, chopped

4 cups vegetable broth

2 tablespoons nutritional yeast

½ teaspoon white pepper

½ teaspoon sea salt

1 bay leaf

1 cup plain yogurt (soy or dairy)

1. In a large stock pot, sauté onion in olive oil.

2. Add remaining ingredients, bring to a boil.

3. Reduce heat to a simmer. Simmer approximately 30 minutes until potatoes and cauliflower are tender.

4. Remove bay leaf.

5. Purée soup in blender.

PER SERVING Calories: 119 • Fat: 3.5 g • Carbohydrates: 18 g • Protein: 4.5 g • Sodium: 239 mg • Fiber: 2 g

The White "Green" Vegetable

The saying "eat your green vegetables" should have the amendment—"and cauliflower." This late-season nutritional powerhouse is a cruciferous vegetable; it's in the same family as broccoli, cabbage, and kale. It has high levels of vitamin C and significant amounts of vitamin B6, folate, and dietary fiber.

Broccoli and Quinoa Casserole

This dish is genuine comfort food with a great consistency for a younger child, but it will please the rest of the family as well. By combining the cooked ingredients without an added baking step, the dish remains very tender and easy for little ones to manage.

INGREDIENTS | SERVES 6

1 cup creamy corn soup

½ cup shredded Cheddar cheese (dairy or soy)

1 large bunch of broccoli

3 cups cooked quinoa

Is Quinoa a Grain?

Although quinoa looks like a grain and cooks like a grain, it is not a true cereal grain. It is actually the seeds of the chenopodium or goosefoot plant. Its relatives include beets, spinach, and Swiss chard.

1. In a small saucepan, heat soup over medium-high heat. Add cheese and stir until melted. Set aside.

2. Cut broccoli into small florets and steam until tender. Combine quinoa, cheese sauce, and broccoli in a serving bowl or casserole dish.

PER SERVING Calories: 280 • Fat: 7.5 g • Carbohydrates: 45 g • Protein: 12 g • Sodium: 109 mg • Fiber: 7 g

Take-Along Cereal Snack

Because raisins can be a choking hazard for children under the age of three, dehydrated fruits step in to create a tasty nutritious snack.

INGREDIENTS | SERVES 9

3 cups O-type cereal

1 cup dried, diced apples

½ cup dried strawberry pieces

1. Combine all ingredients.

2. Store in an airtight container or bag

PER SERVING Calories: 57 • Fat: 0.5 g • Carbohydrates: 13 g • Protein: 1.5 g • Sodium: 77 mg • Fiber: 2 g

PB and B Wrap

Prepare this quick-and-easy wrap first thing in the morning.
If prepared the night before, it is going to be soggy!

INGREDIENTS | SERVES 1

1 whole-wheat wrap

2 tablespoons trans-fat-free peanut butter

2 teaspoons honey

Small ripe banana

A High-Energy Way to Start the Day

Whole-wheat wrap, peanut butter, and banana hits all of the necessary food groups first thing in the morning. Students will be able to give their full concentration to those first few classes of the day. Whole-wheat bread or a whole-wheat roll can be substituted for the wrap.

1. Spread peanut butter and honey onto wrap.

2. Mash banana. Spread onto wrap.

3. Pull up one side of the wrap, about ⅓ of the way, and fold over.

4. Wrap both sides in, and close the top.

PER SERVING Calories: 363 • Fat: 17 g • Carbohydrates: 46 g • Protein: 11 g • Sodium: 171 mg • Fiber: 6 g

Funny Face Pizza

Just a cute way to get the children involved in making their pizza—including those great vegetables, too!

INGREDIENTS | SERVES 4

1 prepared pizza crust (preferably whole wheat)

Nonstick cooking spray

1 (24-ounce) jar spaghetti or pizza sauce

2 cups shredded low-fat mozzarella cheese

Oregano, parsley, pepper, and garlic to taste

4 large carrots, grated

1 black olive

1 cup steamed broccoli florets

1 thin slice red pepper

2 round zucchini slices

1. Preheat oven to 350°F.

2. Lay out pizza crust on a large piece of aluminum foil, sprayed with nonstick cooking spray.

3. Cover pizza crust with tomato sauce, mozzarella cheese, and spices.

4. Decorate with vegetables using grated carrots for hair and eyebrows. Use an olive for the nose and broccoli florets for the eyes. Use red pepper slice for the mouth, and zucchini for the cheeks; or choose different vegetable favorites and use your imagination.

5. Cook pizza according to package directions.

PER SERVING Calories: 252 • Fat: 15 g • Carbohydrates: 30 g • Protein: 18 g • Sodium: 278 mg • Fiber: 5 g

Brave Bean Burritos

*A quick dinner for all—family members can assemble the burritos themselves—
and in 10 minutes, dinner is ready. Add a big fruit salad and voila!*

INGREDIENTS | SERVES 4

4 corn tortillas

2 cups canned black beans, drained

½ cup prepared salsa (optional spice
    level)

½ cup romaine lettuce, chopped finely

½ cup tomatoes, chopped finely

2 ounces low-fat Cheddar cheese,
    shredded

1. Warm tortillas and roll up in aluminum foil.

2. When ready to serve, fill each tortilla equally with
   beans, salsa, lettuce, tomato, and cheese and close
   the burrito.

3. Warm in microwave about 30 seconds until beans are
   hot and cheese is melted.

PER SERVING Calories: 342 • Fat: 4 g • Carbohydrates: 61 g •
Protein: 27 g • Sodium: 223 mg • Fiber: 16 g

Anatomy of a Burrito

As is, this recipe uses black beans; however, kidney beans or white beans or even fat-free refried beans offer great variety. Of course, the spice level of the salsa can be altered; the vegetables that go inside the tortilla can also be different. Lettuce and tomato are the norm, but how about raw mushrooms, sliced colored peppers, jalapeños, shaved carrots, or cucumbers? Cheeses add some protein and calcium—offer the children's favorite low-fat varieties: Monterrey jack, Cheddar, and so on. This dish makes the crowd roar for more!

Grilled Marinated Mahi-Mahi

This recipe is easy, and it's delicious with tilapia, baja, or salmon as well.
The longer it marinates, the better the flavor.

INGREDIENTS | SERVES 6

2 lemons, juiced
2 medium oranges, juiced
Lemon and orange zest (from above)
2 tablespoons brown sugar
1½–2 pounds mahi-mahi

1. Prepare the marinade by blending the lemon and orange juice, lemon and orange zest, and brown sugar in shallow dish.

2. Place the fish into the marinade and refrigerate for a minimum of 2 hours.

3. Grill fish until opaque inside.

PER SERVING Calories: 119 • Fat: 2 g • Carbohydrates: 6 g • Protein: 18 g • Sodium: 48 mg • Fiber: 0 g

CHAPTER 13

Healthy Eating/
Breaking Bad Habits

The best way to achieve your goals is to learn to "eat for energy," focusing on what you should be eating instead of what you shouldn't. Sometimes people don't even notice they aren't consuming as many processed foods as they did in the past. When your body is getting the nutrition it needs, it works more efficiently and doesn't have as many cravings for refined carbohydrates. The trick is sustaining a positive environment whenever you eat. Don't go too long without eating or consume too many "empty" calories. Healthy eating keeps you from feeling deprived. This chapter will support you in building more positive relationships with foods and help you release negative ideas you've had in the past.

A Healthy Start

After twelve hours without nourishment, your body needs a fresh supply in the morning. Your blood glucose needs replenishment so it can furnish the rest of your body with energy. Your brain, especially, needs glucose, as it has no capacity to store it. Eating breakfast aids your concentration, your ability to problem solve, your strength, and your endurance. What's more, intake of nutrients in the morning helps to regulate the appetite throughout the day, increasing your chances of meeting your daily nutritional requirements.

Breakfast is especially important for kids. A healthy breakfast improves overall cognitive skills, including memory, which gives them an edge in test-taking, attendance, and class participation. Kids who skip breakfast tend to be disinterested, irritable, and lack the focus needed to succeed in class. And because a large chunk of their daily nutrients is missing, they tend to visit the school nurse more often.

Helping children develop a good breakfast habit is one of the best ways parents can ensure lifelong success for their offspring.

FACT

The Massachusetts School Nutrition Task Force reports a study in which students participating in school breakfast programs had decreased trips to the school nurse, as well as increased math and reading scores, improved behavior, and attendance.

If that weren't enough to convince you to eat your breakfast, know that people who skip breakfast tend to be heavier. Hunger builds up as lunch approaches, and suddenly food is necessary, in any form. In this situation, it is common to throw caution to the wind and eat the first thing that presents itself. Eating too much of the wrong foods is often the result. Although the day is half over, the daily nutrient intake is far from half complete.

What's Your Excuse?

The general excuse for skipping the first meal of the day is lack of time. Busy lifestyles do not have to preclude health. You can eat a healthy breakfast in ten minutes or less if you plan for it. A bowl of cereal, a piece of fruit, yogurt, and/or slice of whole-wheat toast is adequate.

Some people complain that breakfast upsets their stomachs. Try to eat a small bit of fruit or bland toast each day, then slowly increase your intake as your system grows accustomed to it. It is possible that you have simply been choosing the wrong morning food for your sensitive stomach. You may also want to pack yourself a small breakfast snack, such as a nutrition bar or a piece of fruit, to eat later in the morning, when your stomach is less sensitive.

What Is a Healthy Breakfast?

In general you want to eat foods of high nutritional value in the morning. Avoid sugary cereals, which have few nutrients. They raise your blood sugar quickly, but then drop it way down so you feel hungry again within an hour. Fast food, too, should be avoided, as it is similarly short on nutrients and generally contains excessive fat. Low-fat, low-sugar, high-fiber foods are the way to go. These foods help maintain your blood sugar level for hours and start your day with healthy nutrient intake.

Skipping Meals

Food is fuel. You need it for energy. When you don't eat, you lose energy. It's that simple. But today busy people think they do not always have time for meals. Unfortunately, it is almost impossible to get your daily recommended nutrients if you don't eat—you can't just take vitamin supplements.

The daily nutrients are vital to the healthy functioning of all parts of your body. And although you may not notice when your body is running well, you certainly will notice when it starts to break down.

Good daily nutrition is the easiest way to achieve health and optimal performance. If you're not an Olympic athlete, you may wonder what optimal performance means for you. Brain function, cognitive reasoning, attentiveness, memory, and moods are all affected by nutrition. The things you can't see, including a healthy immune system, are directly related to what you eat as well. Your body needs a constant flow of energy to run smoothly, and eating regularly is crucial to achieving that goal.

Controlling Portion Size

Hefty portions are another big contributor to overeating. Nutritional guidelines give you ample information regarding portions, but they can be a little intimidating. Visions of scales and measuring cups scare people away, and they go back to eating as much as they want. Unfortunately, when you combine large portions with speed eating, bingeing, and poor nutrition overall, the results are devastating.

This is not to suggest that measuring your food is not useful. But you don't need a lab coat and beakers to control your portion size. A simple frame of reference is all you need. In general, most portions should resemble the palm of your hand. (Just the palm, not the fingers.) This is a good reference because everyone's palm is different, enabling you to adjust for variations in age and sex.

Don't serve food "family style." Placing large dishes of food on the table encourages overeating. Worse than that, family style can set up competition for the last piece, which results in speed eating (and sibling disputes).

QUESTION

What is family style?
Family-style service refers to setting large serving dishes on the table. Dishes are passed from person to person, each serving him- or herself. It provides the opportunity for second and third helpings, which means overeating. Instead, put the food on the plates in the kitchen, each with the intended portion.

One last trick to eating less is to serve food on a smaller plate. Your eyes are definitely part of your eating experience. Seeing a tiny piece of food on a huge plate starts the meal off with disappointment.

Caffeine and Alcohol

Except for water, coffee is the world's most consumed beverage. And wine grapes are the world's most abundant crop. But neither of these beverages, though they have significant cultural, social, and historical heritage, offer much nutritional value. Caffeine is a stimulant, and alcohol is a depressant. Both of them alter the way your body functions, and both, when taken in excess, are damaging.

Caffeine

Caffeine is a naturally occurring substance found in the coffee bean, cocoa bean, kola nut, and tea leaf. Taken as a mild stimulant, caffeine increases body temperature, heart rate, and blood pressure. It restricts blood vessels to the brain, which prevents sleep, and causes the release of adrenaline, which makes you alert.

When abused, caffeine causes anxiety, stomach irritation, headaches, and insomnia. What's worse, it is addictive. People who consume more than 300 milligrams a day (about three cups of coffee) will suffer withdrawal symptoms when cut off from their supply. Symptoms include fatigue, depression, irritability, jitters, and headaches as blood vessels in the brain dilate. Additionally, caffeine is a diuretic, flushing your body of fluids. This makes caffeinated beverages a poor choice as fluid replacements for water.

FACT

In addition to being present in your favorite beverages, caffeine can also be found in some medications. Medicine for migraines often includes caffeine, which makes the drug work quickly. Caffeine is sometimes used to counteract drowsiness caused by certain medications, such as antihistamines.

Caffeine is not stored in the body, so its effects are not permanent. It's impact can be felt ten to fifteen minutes after ingestion, and the effect lasts two to three hours. Tolerance for caffeine varies, but most adults should limit intake to 200–300 milligrams per day. One cup of coffee is about 90 milligrams, and sodas average around 40 milligrams.

When cutting back on caffeine, it's best to go slowly. Limit your caffeinated soda and tea intake, and switch your coffee to half-caffeinated. Take heart in knowing that your headaches will disappear in a week or two.

Alcohol

Alcohol was first valued as a way to purify water. But its mind-altering and addictive properties soon became apparent. Alcohol is not in and of itself nutritious, and though certain forms may contain healthful properties, these are negligible in comparison to the damage alcohol does.

Regularly consuming more than the recommended two drinks per day maximum (one for women) raises your chance of high blood pressure, stroke, and certain cancers, including liver, colon, esophageal, mouth, and breast cancer in women. Alcohol promotes dehydration, and it impairs muscle coordination, reflexes, reaction time, and balance. In addition, heavy consumption commonly results in malnutrition and weight gain. Although it does not contain many nutrients, alcohol does have about seven calories for every gram. The calories replace those that would otherwise be consumed by nutritious foods, and alcohol inhibits the functions of many nutrients that are consumed. Like all extras in your diet, alcohol should be used in moderation.

Common Dieting Mistakes

The most common dieting mistakes include focusing on dieting rather than on your diet. Dieting is a temporary plan to promote weight loss or meet a specific nutritional need. If you do not make actual changes in your behavior while following a diet, you won't enjoy long-term success. People tend to miss many of the messages their bodies are trying to send them, which increases their chances of slipping back into old behaviors toward the end of a diet. They don't learn from their experience. They take an all or nothing approach and don't give themselves credit for each step they took toward reaching their goals. Give yourself credit for what you've accomplished in creating your own healthy lifestyle.

Smart Snacking

Contrary to popular belief, snacking can be part of a healthful eating plan. Choosing snacks wisely can help fuel your body between meals, give you an energy boost, and add to your total intake of essential nutrients for the day.

Snacking can also take the edge off hunger between meals. The longer you wait between meals, the more you tend to eat at the next meal. Leaving only about three to four hours between meals is ideal for controlling blood sugar levels. The key to smart snacking is choosing the right types and amounts of food. Mindless snacking or nibbling on high-fat, high-calorie foods can lead to unwanted and empty calories.

QUESTION

Can eating smaller meals more than three times a day be part of a healthy diet?
Yes. Eating small meals means eating smaller portion meals throughout the day, with the same goals of variety, balance, and moderation. For healthful grazing, make sure you still get your needed number of servings from all of the food groups. Balance the foods you eat, and eat smaller portions.

To make snacking a healthy part of your diet, try these tips:

- Choose snacks that are low in fat and nutrient rich.
- Make snacks part of your eating plan for the day instead of thinking of them as an extra.
- Make snacking a conscious activity.
- Plan and eat snacks well ahead of mealtime.
- Eat snacks in smaller portions, not meal-size ones.

Try some of these smart snacks as part of your healthy eating plan:

- ½ bagel with peanut butter
- Raw vegetables with low-fat or fat-free dressing
- Fruit yogurt topped with low-fat granola cereal
- Low-fat cottage cheese topped with fresh fruit
- Fresh fruit
- Light microwave popcorn
- Pita bread stuffed with fresh veggies and low-fat dressing
- Low-fat string cheese

- Whole-grain cereal and fat-free milk
- Vegetable juice

Hunger Versus Cravings

Is it a craving, or are you really hungry? You first need to understand the difference between a physical food craving—or actual hunger—and an emotional food craving. Cravings can be caused by either physical or psychological needs. Emotional cravings or eating triggers are usually caused by psychological needs, whereas hunger is a biological function of the body's real need for food. Emotional cravings can lead to bingeing. Learn to listen to your body, and understand what it is trying to tell you.

Trust yourself to know whether you are craving a food for emotional reasons or if your body is truly hungry. Giving in to too many cravings can lead to overeating, unhealthy eating, and weight gain. Healthy eating means eating when you are truly hungry and eating until you are satisfied. It is being able to choose healthy foods, but not being so restrictive that you miss out on foods you really enjoy.

You can use many techniques to distinguish between biological and emotional cravings. A physical craving has the following qualities:

- You are physiologically hungry.
- The craving does not go away if you try to wait it out.
- The craving intensifies over time.
- Nothing you do will take away the craving except the craved food.

An emotional craving, on the other hand, looks like this:

- You are not physiologically hungry.
- The craving goes away if you wait it out.
- The craving does not intensify over time; the emotion does.
- Doing something else satisfies the real need, and the craving disappears.

Hunger Signals

Being aware of your body's physical hunger signals helps give you the confidence to satisfy your food cravings. Hunger signals can come from your stomach informing you that it is empty or from your brain informing you that it is lacking an energy supply. Signals from your stomach may include growls, pangs, or hollow feelings. Signals from your brain may include fogginess, lack of concentration, headache, or fatigue. If you still are not sure whether you are truly hungry, try using the following Hunger/Fullness Rating Scale.

▼ **Hunger/Fullness Rating Scale**

10	Absolutely, positively stuffed
9	So full that it hurts
8	Very full and bloated
7	Starting to feel uncomfortable
6	Slightly overeaten
5	Perfectly comfortable
4	First signals that your body needs food
3	Strong signals to eat
2	Very hungry, irritable
1	Extreme hunger, dizziness

If you are at level 5 or above, you are not hungry and your body does not physically need food. If you are craving a food, it is emotional, not physical. If you are at level 3 or 4, your body is telling you that it needs some food, and your cravings are physical. If you are at level 1 or 2, your body is too hungry and definitely physically needs food. If you wait until you get to this level you are so hungry that you will probably overeat or eat something that is not healthy.

The best time to eat is at level 3 or 4. At this stage you are experiencing physical hunger, and your body is telling you that you need food. You still have enough control to eat healthful foods and manage your portion sizes.

Craving Solutions

When you are craving foods, determine whether the craving is physical or emotional. Once you have discovered why you want to eat, you can take action. If you determine it is emotional, take steps to try to dissolve your craving in some other way than giving in to the food. For instance, binge-ing or emotional cravings can be due to stress. Stress reduction techniques might include taking a long hot bath, going for a walk, relaxation exercises, meditation, or yoga.

Drink a glass of water before giving in to a craving. Sometimes when you think you're hungry, you're really just thirsty. If you are not only truly hungry but overly hungry, eat something healthy, such as carrot sticks or an apple, instead of the junk food you may be craving. That may fill you up enough to disperse unhealthy food cravings. Use the ten-minute rule. When you crave something, wait ten minutes for the craving to subside. Another option is to satisfy your craving with a very small portion of the food you are craving.

ALERT

Never consume fewer than 1,200 calories a day when trying to lose weight. Below 1,200 calories, your body cannot obtain the proper amount of nutrients required for optimal health. Also, lowering your calories too much can slow down your metabolism, or the rate at which your body burns calories, making it harder to lose and easier to gain the weight back.

Studies suggest that completely avoiding certain foods can make them irresistible and make you crave them even more. The result is that you usu-ally will give in to the craving, overindulge, and then feel guilty for letting it happen. If you are truly physically hungry, eat (in moderation, of course). Keep in mind that you are hungrier on some days than others. So when you're really, truly hungry, it's fine to eat more. Remember that one meal does not define healthy eating habits. What you eat over the course of a day, or over several days, does. Healthy eating is flexible. Giving in to a craving, in moderation, can be part of a healthy eating pattern, so long as it does not get out of hand.

Eating Triggers

Many things can trigger your desire to eat. The aroma of food, the sight of a favorite food, a commercial on television, or just knowing there are sweets in the house. The habit of eating while watching television can make television an eating trigger. Recognizing what triggers eating or cravings is the first step to controlling them.

Keeping a food diary can help identify your eating triggers. This can help you notice when you eat and what you are doing or thinking when you have a craving. If you find that sitting in front of the television is a major trigger for cravings, do something when you watch TV. Knit, write letters, or pay your bills, for instance. Do something that will keep your hands busy and keep your mind off food. If boredom is a trigger, make a list of alternate activities, such as talking to a friend, taking a walk, or washing the car. When you get bored and want to eat, read your list of other options instead.

The key is to learn to recognize cravings and triggers, and then to set up an action plan to deal with them. Cravings are a normal part of our lives, and a healthy eating plan will enable you to cope in a sensible manner.

CHAPTER 14

Vegetarian, Vegan, Organic

A plant-based diet offers many health benefits; however, it can be extremely challenging to sustain a nutritionally complete diet without eating animal products. Lean protein sources can be hard to come by, and choosing nutritious meat alternatives can be confusing. Do your research and determine your individual goals. Which foods do you choose to eat? No meat or fish? No animal products of any kind? Lacto-ovo vegetarian? Vegan? Macrobiotic? Perhaps there isn't a term that fits you exactly, and that is okay! What's important is that you feel comfortable and confident with your food choices. This chapter will help you create a well-balanced diet that suits you.

What Is a Healthy Vegetarian Diet?

As most experts agree, including the American Dietetic Association, a balanced vegetarian diet does provide all a person's recommended daily nutrients. But there's a catch: not all vegetarians practice the same form of vegetarianism, so no one diet fits all. A new vegetarian's best bet is to become familiar with the key nutrients and where to find them. It may also be worth consulting a registered dietitian or a nutritionist to get the pertinent nutritional information. If you make that choice, be sure to select someone who is well trained and who has had experience in counseling vegetarians and in planning a vegetarian menu.

With knowledge of body chemistry and an understanding of food science, that person can take a medical history, and then question you about what you have been eating, why you are making the dietary change, and what your food likes and dislikes are. He or she will know your age and probably ask about your activity level—if you exercise regularly and are fairly active, your nutritional needs will be higher. Then you two can plan what your meals should include, so you can buy, cook, and eat the most wholesome foods.

ESSENTIAL

Food pyramids tell the tale: Click inside the USDA pyramid at *www .mypyramid.gov/pyramid/index.html*, where, if you omit the meats, the USDA pyramid helps you plan your meals. For more information, refer to the USDA's vegetarian tips at *www.mypyramid.gov/tips_re-sources/vegetarian_diets.html*.

Whether you consult a dietitian or just map out your own vegetarian plan, you need to know some basics. Key nutrients include protein; vitamins D, B12, and A; and minerals iron, calcium, and zinc. You will also need a source of omega-3 fatty acids, important for preventing heart disease. Fish and fish oils are the most abundant natural source. Unless you are an lacto-ovo vegetarian who eats eggs from hens fed a diet that contains omega-3 fatty acids or a pescatarian-vegetarian who eats fish, you'll need to find another source. Other good sources include flaxseed oil and such vegetable oils as olive and canola.

Study the Oldways Preservation Trust Vegetarian Diet Pyramid and write your shopping list accordingly. The majority of your food choices and the basics for a sound vegetarian diet will come from the largest food groups: fruits and vegetables, whole grains, and legumes.

If you are a lacto-ovo vegetarian, you should include moderate amounts of dairy products and eggs. For added calcium and protein, include soy foods such as soymilk and soy "meat" analogs—and be sure to incorporate vegetable oils. Meat-like soy products, such as sausages, bacon, ground beef, and ham, are readily available and add variety to a greens-and-grains-based diet. These are lower in fat and calories than their meat counterparts, an important consideration if you have made the vegetarian switch to lose weight or for reasons related to heart health. At the top of your pyramid are the foods you'll eat the least: whole eggs and sweets.

Because vegans eat no dairy products or eggs, their diets are often deficient in and even lack some basics, such as calcium from milk and vitamin B12, a nutrient found exclusively in animal proteins. Vegans may need to add dietary supplements to meet all their nutrient needs. Consider fortified foods such as soymilk with added nutrients and fortified breakfast cereals to your daily menu plans.

As you see, you can eat well and live a healthy vegetarian life—but you must learn what your body needs to stay healthy. Becoming a vegetarian is not just a matter of abstaining from meat. It requires understanding what you need to eat for optimal health and planning accordingly.

A Vegetarian's Food Plan

As most experts agree, eating the vegetarian way can provide all the necessary nutrients. But as you have learned, there's no single diet and no single source for every nutrient. The key to your success is combining foods from different groups and then getting enough calories to meet your age and activity level.

To get it right, say the experts at the Oldways Preservation Trust, you'll need several daily servings from the food groups—fruits and vegetables, whole grains, and legumes—at the base of their pyramid. But you should be sure to eat moderate servings from all the food levels, and drink enough water each day to stay healthy. Make sure your diet contains the appropriate balance of carbohydrates, fats, and proteins.

Processed Foods

The Oldways Preservation Trust staff also stresses that you should avoid processed foods and select, instead, the whole foods that are complete as nature intended them. Processed grains, sugars, and flours are often stripped of their natural nutrients. Even when vitamins and minerals are added back in later—a process called "enriching," which means the nutrients lost during refining are added back in to enrich the product—the total effect is never the same.

White rice, for example, may cook faster and have a more adaptable taste, but by stripping away the outer bran layer, the rice grains lose much of their beneficial fiber and minerals. As proof, one cup of brown rice contains 3.5 grams of fiber. One cup of white rice contains less than one gram. Even enriching white rice doesn't make up the difference in the loss of fiber and minerals.

Another confusing term for consumers is fortifying, and many of today's foods are fortified with added vitamins and minerals. Fortifying milk with vitamin D is one example; adding folic acid to specific foods is another. Enriching means putting back into a refined food nutrients lost during processing; fortifying means perhaps putting back lost nutrients, but also adding others that may not occur naturally in a particular food.

Processing or refining plant foods can also destroy the complex plant chemicals known as phytonutrients, or phytochemicals. Many of these naturally occurring chemicals have health-supporting benefits and have been consumed for centuries for their antioxidant, anti-inflammatory, and anti-carcinogenic properties. Considering that salicin, extracted from the white willow tree, has long been recognized as a painkiller and the basis for today's aspirin, it's easy to understand why unprocessed fruits and vegetables can be your body's best friends.

FACT

According to the USDA, phytonutrients may act as antioxidants, cause cancer cells to die, repair DNA damaged from smoking, and improve the body's immune response.

Daily Needs and Food Sources

According to Katherine Tallmadge, a spokesperson for the American Dietetic Association and a practicing nutritionist, the daily diet program presented here, based on the ADA guidelines, should guide vegetarians to eat right.

MILK AND MILK ALTERNATIVES GROUP: SIX TO EIGHT SERVINGS DAILY

- ½ cup milk, yogurt, or fortified soymilk
- ¾ ounce natural cheese
- ½ to 1 cup cottage cheese
- ¼ cup calcium-set tofu
- 1 cup cooked dry beans, such as soy, cannellini, pinto, navy, Great Northern, kidney, and black beans
- ¼ cup shelled almonds
- 3 tablespoons sesame tahini or almond butter
- 1 cup cooked or 2 cups raw bok choy, Chinese cabbage, broccoli, collards, kale, or okra
- 1 tablespoon blackstrap molasses
- 5 figs

DRY BEANS, NUTS, SEEDS, EGGS, AND MEAT SUBSTITUTES GROUP: TWO TO THREE SERVINGS DAILY

- 1 cup cooked dry beans, lentils, or peas
- 2 cups soymilk
- ½ cup tofu or tempeh
- 2 ounces vegetarian "meats" or soy cheese
- 2 eggs or 4 egg whites
- ¼ cup nuts or seeds
- 3 tablespoons nut or seed butters

FRUIT GROUP: TWO TO FOUR SERVINGS DAILY

- ¾ cup juice
- ¼ cup dried fruit
- ½ cup chopped raw fruit
- ½ cup canned fruit
- 1 medium-size piece of fruit such as banana, apple, or orange

VEGETABLE GROUP: THREE TO FIVE SERVINGS DAILY

- ½ cup cooked or chopped raw vegetables
- 1 cup raw, leafy vegetables
- ¾ cup vegetable juice

BREAD, CEREAL, RICE, AND PASTA GROUP: SIX TO ELEVEN SERVINGS DAILY

- 1 slice (1 ounce) bread
- ½ small bagel, bun, or English muffin (about 1 ounce)
- 1 ounce ready-to-eat cereal
- 2 tablespoons wheat germ
- ½ cup cooked (1 ounce dry) grains, cereal, rice, or pasta

FATS, OILS, SWEETS: USE SPARINGLY

- Candy, butter, dairy fats, solid margarine (high in trans fats)

Do Raw Foods Count?

Some vegetarians follow a raw-foods diet, but they should take special care with the fruits and vegetables they eat. According to the Centers for Disease Control (CDC), raw animal foods—including eggs and raw milk—may contain pathogens. But CDC scientists point out that any raw food exposed to a contaminated food source can contain pathogens.

Likewise, pathogens can readily contaminate raw fruits and vegetables, particularly if these were processed in unsanitary conditions, were fertilized with contaminated manure, or were washed for packing in unclean water. Even unpasteurized fruit juices may be unsafe if made from contaminated fresh fruits. Washing whole fresh produce at home may diminish but not totally eliminate any pathogens.

Achieving the Switch to Vegetarianism

If you have decided that vegetarianism makes sense for you and your lifestyle, you may want to start slowly, learning what you need to eat and trying out the various vegetarian options in your market. Veggies and fruits are one thing, but what about all those different tofu and soy products? How do they fit in?

Plan a week's worth of menus, basing your main dishes on ones you love but switching, say, the beef meatballs for vegetarian ones. Or if you are a chili-head, why not create some really appealing meatless chilis? For that meaty texture, add taco-seasoned soy ground meat with plenty of beans and salsa for a satisfying entrée.

If cheese is your secret passion and you're a vegan, try shredded or sliced soy cheeses in your favorite recipes. These soy products taste and look like meats and dairy cheese, so you won't feel deprived of your favorite foods. Even if you get derailed along the way, and keep a few meats and seafood in your menus, you will feel you're on your way to making the great vegetarian leap.

Answering the Naysayers

Once you've started on the path, and friends and family see that you've changed how and what you eat, you may face criticism or teasing. As the Vegetarian Resource Group advises, point out to people that vegetarianism is becoming increasingly popular. Add that eating a meat-free diet is a personal choice you've made for the following reason or reasons, then list them.

You might also win over others to your way of cooking, living, and eating by preparing delicious vegetarian meals, or at the very least, taking friends and family along when you eat at a vegetarian restaurant. They may be in for a real surprise, especially when they total up the bill and see how reasonable vegetarian food costs can be.

Vegetarian Restaurants

Back in the 1970s, the Moosewood Restaurant in Ithaca, New York, launched a revolutionary restaurant movement by creating and serving outstanding all-vegetarian dishes, inspiring future generations of restaurateurs to follow in their vegetarian footsteps. Since then, not surprisingly, more all-veg restaurants are opening their doors to an influx of new customers. A national Restaurant Association poll from 2001 showed that 1.5 percent of entrées are vegetarian; about eight out of ten restaurants offer vegetarian entrées. Many upscale eateries with white-tablecloth manners have taken up the vegetarian challenge and offer vegetarian options. Even some fast-food outlets are getting in on the act.

Although not all cities and towns feature vegetarian restaurants, in many communities with an Indian or Chinese population, consumers can readily find South Indian or Chinese Buddhist vegetarian restaurants; these still account for the majority of vegetarian establishments. It's not uncommon for mainstream restaurants to acknowledge that their customer base more frequently requests vegetarian entrées. At least one website offers restaurants a restaurant starter kit that tells them what vegetarian consumers look for and how to cook it for them.

Staying Veg

Welcome to the world of vegetarian meals. You've walked the path successfully, but now you ask yourself, Can I stick to the plan? Of course, but if you feel you need family support, ask for it. Treat yourself to vegetarian cookbooks so that your mealtimes don't become routine and your food boring. Continue to learn about this new lifestyle, perhaps monitoring any health or energy changes you note. That way, you'll feel positive about the choices you've made and perhaps inspire others, too.

Vegan Nutrition

Being vegan means cutting out all animal products from your diet. You may wonder where vegans get their protein with no meat or even dairy in their diet. Despite a national obsession with protein, most Americans eat much more than recommended, and deficiency in vegans is rare. Professional body builders and pregnant women aside, most vegans easily meet their daily requirement of protein (and most omnivores exceed it exponentially). Pay special attention, however, to your zinc, vitamin D, iron, and calcium intake, and foremost, vitamin B12.

If you are pregnant, you'll need to plan adequately to obtain all the nutrients you need—not just protein. Consult with your doctor about this. And, as most body builders already know, the timing of protein consumption coupled with the stress of lifts is more important than whether that protein is plant or animal based.

Though not readily supplied by a vegan diet, vitamin D is easily obtained from sunlight. Step outside for a few minutes a day and you're set for vitamin D. Make sure your vegan kids do the same. If you happen to be a vegan living in places where sunshine is limited, it's best to rely on a supplement or fortified foods, such as fortified orange juice or soy milk.

Similarly, many soy foods are fortified with calcium, another important nutrient for dairy-free folks. Broccoli, tofu, tahini, almonds, and dark leafy greens also provide a good natural source. To build strong bones, you need exercise as well as calcium, so vegan or not, diet is only half the equation.

ALERT

Before you pour that glass of orange juice or soy milk, shake it up! The calcium in these drinks tends to settle at the bottom of the carton, so to get the best bone-boosting effect, shake before you drink. If you're a heavy smoker or coffee drinker, consider taking a supplement, as cigarettes and coffee inhibit absorption of several nutrients.

When it comes to iron, most vegans and vegetarians actually get more than omnivores. Lentils, chickpeas, tahini, and, once again, those dark leafy greens such as spinach and kale are good vegan sources of iron.

Noticing a pattern? Dark leafy green vegetables are one of the most nutrient-rich foods on the planet. Find ways to include kale, spinach, or other greens in your diet by snipping them into pasta sauces and casseroles, or include a few spinach leaves along with your other salad greens.

Fish oils and fish such as salmon are often touted as a source of healthy omega-3 fatty acids, but vegetarians and vegans can obtain these from flaxseeds and flaxseed oil, as well as walnuts or hemp seeds.

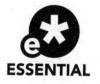

ESSENTIAL

Flaxseed oil is rich in omega-3s and has a sweet and nutty flavor. Never use it as a cooking oil, however, as the heat destroys the healthy fats and creates unhealthy free radicals. Instead, add a teaspoonful of flax oil to your favorite salad dressing, or drizzle it over already cooked dishes for your daily quotient of omega-3s. Look for a brand that is cold-pressed and store chilled to keep it fresh.

Vitamin B12 cannot reliably be obtained from vegan foods. Deficiencies of this important nutrient are admittedly rare, and, if you're eating vegan meals only occasionally, you don't need to worry. Vegetarians will absorb B12 from food sources, but long-term vegans, and pregnant and breast-feeding women, in particular, need a reliable source. Take a supplement and eat fortified foods, such as nutritional yeast. Because the body needs very little B12, and it can be stored for years, some people claim a supplement is not needed, or suggest that omnivores are more likely to be deficient in a variety of nutrients, and thus the B12 issue for vegans is grossly overblown. Although this last argument may be true, the bottom line, according to most experts, is to take a supplement. Better safe than sorry.

The Truth about Protein

In 1971, Frances Moore Lappé wrote a book that revolutionized the relationship thousands of Americans had with their plates, effectively launching vegetarianism into the public consciousness. *Diet for a Small Planet* continues to be a widely read and cited book today. Much to the chagrin of generations of vegetarians, however, it was the beginning of a myth still oft retold. This is the myth of "protein combining," or the idea that plant sources provide "incomplete" proteins whereas meats provide "complete" proteins.

FACT

Quinoa, soy, and hemp seeds are vegan powerhouses for protein, as they contain the highest amount of all nine essential amino acids. Hemp seeds are also high in omega-3 and omega-6 essential fatty acids.

Lappé theorized that in order to digest all nine of the essential amino acids the human body needs to build protein, vegetarians needed to combine foods so as to consume each essential amino acid in one sitting. Whole grains needed to be consumed at the same time as nuts, for example.

The truth is, by eating a variety of foods, you'll have nothing to worry about. Although you do need a full range of amino acids, and some plant-based foods contain more or less of the essentials, Lappé's error was assuming these nine essentials must be consumed at the same meal. Nutritionists, including the American Dietetic Association and the USDA, have since refuted this claim, and even Lappé herself revised her stance in later editions of the book. Your body will store and combine proteins on its own.

If, however, you tend to go weeks eating nothing but bananas and soda, you'll quickly find yourself deficient in more than just protein. But eat a relatively healthy diet and you'll be just fine. According to the American Dietetic Association, "Plant sources of protein alone can provide adequate amounts of the essential and nonessential amino acids, assuming that dietary protein sources from plants are reasonably varied."

Vegan Health Advantages

Although B12 deficiency is a genuine concern, the health advantages of a plant-based diet are endless. The average vegan gets twice as much fiber as most omnivores. A vegan diet is naturally cholesterol free, and is almost guaranteed to lead to marked decreases in cholesterol levels in just two weeks. If lowering your cholesterol naturally is one of your goals, test your levels before and again a few weeks into a vegan diet—and gamble with your skeptical friends, just for fun.

But this is just the tip of the iceberg.

Blood pressure, too, is shown to decrease drastically in a short period of time on a plant-based diet. High blood pressure is a rarely a concern for vegans, and making the switch can decrease your blood pressure in less than two months. No need to give up salt as conventional wisdom dictates—just get rid of the meat and dairy products.

As an added bonus for men (and for women too, really), it's possible that vegans really do make better lovers. High blood pressure, high cholesterol, and particularly the decreased blood flow associated with blocked arteries are common causes leading to erectile dysfunction, and vegans certainly have fewer instances of these symptoms. Sure, a little purple pill can help out for the night, but a vegan diet can help forever!

The fountain of youth may not flow with water after all—it may be full of fruits and veggies.

You do need to eat a balanced diet in order to reap these benefits. After all, French fries and potato chips are animal free, but that doesn't make them healthy. When it comes to vegan nutrition, variety is key. Make sure your protein sources are varied, rather than from just one food group. Eat a rainbow of fruits and veggies, and include green leafy vegetables as often as possible.

The health benefits of reduced animal consumption aren't just personal, they're global as well. The powerful cocktail of hormones and antibiotics pumped into cows and chickens by today's food industry ends up right back in local water supplies and affects everyone, even vegans. All these antibiotics, combined with the cramped conditions on modern farms, lead to dangerous new drug-resistant pathogens and bacterial strains. Swine flu, bird flu, SARS, and mad-cow disease are all traced back to intense animal agriculture practices. Because of our rapidly shrinking planet, the "butterfly effect" is a very real phenomenon: a pig in Mexico sneezed, and a child in Bangkok died.

Getting Started with Veganism

There's no need to toss out all your old cookbooks and family recipes—many of them can provide inspiration for fabulous vegan meals after a few minor tweaks, of course. Most recipes for cookies, muffins, and cakes can be made with nondairy milk, vegan margarine, and a commercial egg replacer. For recipes calling for honey, try an equivalent amount of agave nectar, which is equally lovely in tea and drizzled over vegan pancakes. Store-bought mock ground beef is surprisingly tasty, and textured vegetable protein (TVP) granules provide a meaty texture in dishes such as tacos or chili.

ESSENTIAL

Cooking for omnivores? If your family still insists on eating meat, no need to cook two separate meals. Prepare a bit of meat separately, and add it into only a portion of an otherwise vegan soup, pasta, or casserole.

Take a look at some of your favorite meals. Do you like spaghetti with meatballs? Try a vegetable marinara instead, or grab some ready-made vegetarian meatballs from your grocery store. You can make your favorite chicken noodle soup recipe without the chicken, and omit the beef from your Chinese beef and broccoli, or use seitan as a beef substitute instead. Often, it's the spices, flavors, and textures that make a meal satisfying and nostalgic, not the actual meat.

For the novice chef, restaurants can offer a tasty introduction to new foods. Check your phonebook or the Internet for vegetarian and vegan restaurants in your area. Thai and Chinese restaurants serve up vegan curries and stir-fries, many with an array of mock meats. As a general rule, ethnic restaurants including Mexican (just hold the cheese), Indian, and Middle Eastern places provide more options for vegetarians and vegans than American chains and diners, which may offer little more than a veggie burger as an afterthought.

Creating Amazing Meals

At restaurants, the flavors often come from an overdose of salt, fat, and sometimes MSG. But when cooking at home, you're better off enhancing your foods with flavors that come from nature.

One flavor enhancer unique to vegan cuisine is nutritional yeast. It's a yellowish powder universally loved by vegans for its nutty and cheesy taste, and its ability to add that "je ne sais quoi" to just about any savory dish.

ALERT

Watch out for brewer's yeast, which many well-meaning people insist is the same as nutritional yeast. It's not. Depending on where you live, nutritional yeast may be called "savory yeast flakes" or "nutritional food yeast," but brewer's yeast is something altogether different.

Most chefs agree that sea salt has a superior taste to table salt. Once you've tried sea salt, you'll never go back to regular refined salt, and the trace minerals in sea salt are an added bonus. Similarly, freshly cracked black pepper is always best. Use vegetable broth instead of water whenever possible. Stock up on vegetarian bouillon or powdered vegetable broth, and don't be afraid to use it with a heavy hand in stir-fries, soups, gravies, and casseroles—just about anything savory or spicy.

Fresh herbs and spices are an obvious choice for adding flavor, but their true power comes in their variety and combination. No matter how many spices are on your spice rack, there's always room for one or two more! Most of the spices called for in this book are commonly found, but don't let that limit you. Add garam masala to Indian dishes and smoked Spanish paprika to paellas. Same with fresh herbs. If you can find them, add lemongrass and kaffir lime leaves to your Thai curries.

ESSENTIAL

Got a big bunch of basil? Make your fresh herbs last longer by giving them a quick rinse. Then, wrap your slightly damp herbs in a paper towel. Place the paper towel in a zip-top bag and store in your refrigerator's crisper. They'll keep about ten days this way.

One or two gourmet or unusual ingredients can add pizzazz to an otherwise standard dish. A salad drizzled with champagne vinegar and avocado oil trumps regular vinaigrette any day, and a meatless pasta salad enhanced with sun-dried tomatoes, dried blueberries, or artichoke hearts, for example, is more exciting than a pasta salad with ordinary grilled chicken. The difference between a simple meal and a culinary affair to remember may be just a handful of wasabi-coated macadamia nuts.

When to Choose Organic

In 2002, the USDA label was implemented and replaced private organic labeling programs. A concern arose about the level of standards in the new label after synthetic additive traces were found in products such as baby food. The demand for organic food products has tremendously increased and the industry has expanded to a $20 billion per year business. The label is no longer a guarantee consumers can trust, however. In general, limiting processed foods and purchasing from local farmers is the safest way to consume most of your organic food.

Confusion about whether to buy organic or not in the produce section may be a factor in the lack of organic fruit and vegetable consumption in the United States. According to the USDA Economic Research Service, vegetable consumption has slumped slightly, to 92.2 pounds per person per year in 2008, from a peak of 101 pounds in 1999. The higher cost of organic foods may also overwhelm some consumers. A need existed for a simple tool to help consumers feel confident in their purchases, so The Environmental Working Group has provided the public with their Shopper's Guide to Pesticides, updated in 2010. You can view the guide at *www.foodnews.org*. This is a great resource to for consumers who would like to improve their health.

Which foods make sense to buy organic?

- Meat: beef, pork, chicken, and turkey
- Milk and dairy products
- Eggs
- Baby food
- Juices
- Coffee

The fruits and vegetables found lowest in pesticides, according to the CLEAN 15 from the Environmental Working Group are:

- Onions
- Avocados
- Sweet corn
- Pineapple
- Mangoes
- Sweet peas
- Asparagus
- Kiwi
- Cabbage
- Eggplant
- Cantaloupe
- Watermelon
- Grapefruit
- Sweet potatoes,
- Honeydew melon

Recipes

Cellophane Noodle Salad

In the traditional Thai version of this salad, cooks use fish sauce instead of soy sauce and ground pork, shrimp, and/or chicken for the meat. Thais also are likely to use chiles that they crumble into the bowl. Mighty hot.

INGREDIENTS | SERVES 4

4 ounces cellophane, or bean thread, noodles, softened in hot water for 20 minutes

1 (6-ounce) package soy "chicken" strips, optional

½ cup thinly sliced scallions

½ cup fresh cilantro leaves

1–2 tablespoons crushed red peppers

2 tablespoons lime juice

2 tablespoons soy sauce

1 tablespoon pickled garlic, chopped

Sugar, to taste

1. Drain the soaked and softened noodles and cut them into serving-sized pieces. Put the noodles, "chicken" strips (if using), scallions, cilantro leaves, and crushed red peppers into a serving bowl.

2. Mix together the lime juice, soy sauce, and pickled garlic and toss with the salad ingredients.

PER SERVING Calories: 170 • Fat: 1.5 g • Protein: 9 g • Sodium: 590 mg • Carbohydrates: 32 g • Fiber: 3 g

What Are Cellophane Noodles?

Called "glass," "cellophane," or "bean thread" noodles, this Asian pasta is made from the starch of mung beans. When dried, the noodles are so brittle and tough the cleanest way to cut them is with scissors—they may fly around, so hold them over the sink. They are easier to cut when wet, although they are also somewhat gelatinous. Unless you plan to put the softened noodles in a soup, drain them before using them in other dishes. These are readily available at most well-stocked supermarkets and at Asian markets.

Veggie Frittata

Versatile and adaptable to whichever veggies are in season, this wholesome dish starts the day with a bang, and it makes a good light supper, too. It's also easy to increase quantities to feed larger groups.

INGREDIENTS | SERVES 4

3 tablespoons olive oil

2 red potatoes, diced

6 asparagus spears, trimmed and cut into 2-inch lengths

½ zucchini or yellow summer squash, diced

2 teaspoons minced garlic

1 teaspoon seasoning salt

1 teaspoon smoked paprika

6 large eggs

1 cup shredded Cheddar cheese

½ cup chopped Italian parsley

What's Smoked Paprika?

A Spanish seasoning made from slowly oak-smoked and ground pimentón, a variety of Spanish red pepper, smoked paprika imparts an earthy, woodsy taste to an infinite number of savory dishes. It's readily available in well-stocked supermarkets, specialty food stores, and online mail-order sites.

1. Preheat the broiler.

2. Heat the oil in an 8" or 9" skillet over medium heat. Add the potatoes and sauté for about 3 minutes or until the cubes begin to brown. Add the asparagus, zucchini, garlic, and seasonings and cover the skillet, cooking for 2–3 minutes.

3. Meanwhile, beat the eggs until foamy. Stir in the cheese and parsley and pour the egg mixture over the vegetables. Using a spatula, lift up the edges of the eggs and tip the skillet to all sides, allowing the uncooked eggs to flow underneath the vegetables and to cook.

4. When the eggs are almost firm, slide the skillet under the broiler and cook until the top is bubbly and brown. Serve hot sliced in wedges; the cheese should be melted and runny.

PER SERVING Calories: 350 • Fat: 23 g • Protein: 16 g • Sodium: 430 mg • Carbohydrates: 20 g • Fiber: 2 g

Fruit-and-Cheese Quesadillas

Bland mozzarella is a perfect backdrop for fruit, and you can vary the fruit and jam according to what's seasonally available. These are knife-and-fork quesadillas, too gooey for finger food.

INGREDIENTS | SERVES 4

4 tablespoons strawberry jam

4 (6- to 8-inch) whole-wheat flour tortillas

2 cups shredded mozzarella cheese

1 cup diced fresh strawberries, plus extra for sprinkling

4 tablespoons strawberry yogurt, for garnish

Confectioners' sugar, for dusting

1. Spread 1 tablespoon jam on a tortilla and sprinkle it with ¼ cup mozzarella cheese and ¼ cup diced strawberries. Fold over the tortilla to enclose the filling. Repeat with the remaining tortillas, mozzarella, jam, and strawberries.

2. Spray the skillet with nonstick cooking spray and heat it over medium heat. Cook the quesadillas, one or two at a time, until golden on the bottom, about 3 minutes. Flip over and cook the second side until golden and the cheese has melted.

3. Top each quesadilla with a dollop of yogurt, a sprinkling of strawberries, and a dusting of confectioners' sugar. Serve hot.

PER SERVING Calories: 380 • Fat: 16 g • Protein: 17 g • Sodium: 530 mg • Carbohydrates: 42 g • Fiber: 3 g

Trail Mix Cookies

These chunky cookies will spoil your kids. The total "trail mix" add-ins may range between 3–3¼ cups. You can vary what you add to the mix, of course, but don't go over the total 3¼ cups.

INGREDIENTS | MAKES ABOUT 4 DOZEN COOKIES

1 cup unsalted butter, at room temperature

1½ cups firmly packed brown sugar

1 cup granulated sugar

2 large eggs

2 teaspoons vanilla extract

2½ cups white whole-wheat flour

1 cup all-purpose flour

1 teaspoon baking soda

1 teaspoon salt

¾ cup chocolate chips

¾ cup jelly beans

¾ cup dried papaya cubes

⅓ cup dried cranberries

⅓ cup dried blueberries

⅓ cup pumpkin seeds

What Is Trail Mix?

Long-lasting and very portable, trail mix has become a favorite pick-me-up for people who enjoy rigorous activities such as hiking and camping. The mixture usually consists of such energy-dense foods as nuts, raisins, other dried fruits, chocolate bits, and granola and/or oats—a great energizer for kids! It's called "scroggin" in Australia and New Zealand.

1. Cream together butter and sugars until light and fluffy. Beat in the eggs, one at a time, mixing well after each addition. Stir in the vanilla.

2. Combine the flours, baking soda, and salt, and stir into the butter-egg mixture. Mix until smooth, scraping down the dough from the sides of the bowl. If the dough still feels sticky, stir in extra white whole-wheat flour, a few tablespoons at a time. Combine the trail mix ingredients in a separate bowl and stir them into the dough, making sure to distribute them evenly. Cover the dough with plastic wrap and refrigerate for at least 6 hours or overnight.

3. Preheat the oven to 350°F. Scoop out a heaping tablespoon of dough for each cookie and place the dough on a nonstick cookie sheet. Repeat until the sheet is full, spacing the cookies about 1 inch apart; this should average about 12 cookies per sheet.

4. Bake the cookies for about 10 minutes or until the edges begin to turn brown. Let the cookies cool on the sheet before removing them and baking the next batch. Repeat until all the cookie dough is used up.

PER COOKIE Calories: 150 • Fat: 5 g • Protein: 2 g • Sodium: 55 mg • Carbohydrates: 27 g • Fiber: 2 g

Veggie Quesadillas

Most supermarkets now stock flour tortillas in several flavors, which gives you a chance to use healthier whole-wheat or multigrain options. You might even try a flavored tortilla such as spinach, basil, or sun-dried tomato for a change of pace.

INGREDIENTS | SERVES 6

6 (8-inch) whole-wheat or multigrain tortillas

2½ cups shredded Cheddar cheese

2 cups mixed shredded or cut-up vegetables

½ cup salsa

Which Veggies?

These quesadillas are great vehicles for getting kids to eat their vegetables. Of course, offer their favorites, but why not slip in others, maybe radishes and sprouts? Head to your nearest salad bar and pick out a combination of vegetables—even pitted black olives and a three-bean salad—as fillings. Just make sure the ones you select are shredded or sliced thinly enough to wrap up in the tortilla.

1. Preheat a large skillet or griddle over medium heat and spray it lightly with nonstick cooking spray.

2. Place 1 tortilla on a flat surface and sprinkle it with ½ cup cheese. Put about ⅓ cup vegetables and 2 tablespoons salsa on half of the tortilla and fold it over to close. Place the tortilla on the griddle and heat until the first side turns golden and the cheese melts. Flip over to cook the second side. Repeat with the remaining ingredients, spraying with nonstick cooking spray as needed—don't let the griddle overheat. Cut the quesadillas into serving portions and serve hot.

PER SERVING Calories: 300 • Fat: 16 g • Protein: 16 g • Sodium: 670 mg • Carbohydrates: 27 g • Fiber: 4 g

Taco Pie

This wholesome entrée packs all the kid-favorite flavors of the Southwest into easy-to-serve portions. You can garnish each portion with guacamole, sour cream, chopped black olives, more salsa for an extra kick, and snipped fresh cilantro.

INGREDIENTS | SERVES 6

1 (16-ounce) can pinto beans, drained and rinsed

2 cups shredded Cheddar cheese

1 cup crushed taco chips

½ cup salsa of your choice

½ cup sunflower seeds

2 teaspoons taco seasoning, or to taste

1 (9-inch) deep-dish unbaked pie crust

Boosting Flavors

If your child likes taco flavors, seize the opportunity to introduce other Tex-Mex flavors. Substitute Monterrey jack cheese with jalapeños for more bite, or check out the Hispanic foods section in your grocery store to come up with other flavor options, using tomatillos and different types of salsas.

1. Preheat the oven to 350°F.

2. Combine the beans, cheese, ½ cup taco chips, salsa, sunflower seeds, and taco seasonings. Sprinkle the remaining ½ cup taco chips onto the pie crust. Scoop the bean mixture into the shell, smoothing out the top.

3. Bake for 25–30 minutes or until the filling feels firm. Remove and set aside to cool slightly before slicing to serve. Garnish as desired.

PER SERVING Calories: 440 • Fat: 27 g • Protein: 15 g • Sodium: 730 mg • Carbohydrates: 37 g • Fiber: 6 g

Fiery Indian Potatoes

This unusual potato dish is not for the faint of heart—the chili component can singe your eyebrows. Yet it is a delicious dish and pairs well with thick plain yogurt or as an accompaniment to other vegetarian dishes. Look for the Indian red chili powder at an Indian market; otherwise, use ground cayenne.

INGREDIENTS | SERVES 6

6 large potatoes, peeled and cubed

3 tablespoons vegetable oil, or more as needed

5 dried red chiles, or to taste, crushed

1 tablespoon mustard seeds

1 teaspoon ground turmeric

1 teaspoon red chili powder

Salt and freshly ground black pepper, to taste

1 tablespoon ground coriander

1 cup chopped fresh cilantro, for garnish

1. Steam the potato cubes until just tender. Set aside.

2. Heat the oil in a large skillet or wok, and sauté the potatoes for 2 minutes. Add the chiles, mustard seeds, turmeric, chili powder, salt, and pepper and continue cooking over medium heat, stirring, until the seasonings are well mixed and the potatoes begin to brown. Stir in the coriander, garnish with the cilantro, and serve.

PER SERVING Calories: 370 • Protein: 9 g • Sodium: 30 mg • Fat: 8 g • Carbohydrates: 69 g • Fiber: 9 g

Mediterranean Galette with Goat Cheese

You can add more capers and goat cheese, if you want.

INGREDIENTS | SERVES 6

2 tablespoons olive oil

4 cloves garlic, crushed and chopped

1 onion, diced

1 red bell pepper, seeded and diced

1 (13¾-ounce) can artichoke hearts, drained and quartered

1 sheet puff pastry, thawed

½ cup chopped Niçoise olives

3 tablespoons capers

4 ounces goat cheese, cut into cubes

What Is a Galette?

In France, the word *galette* can mean a flat bread or, as in this case, an open-faced and free-form tart. Fillings may be either sweet or savory.

1. Preheat the oven to 375°F.

2. Heat the oil in a large skillet over medium heat and sauté the garlic and the onion for about 3 minutes. Add the pepper and artichoke hearts and continue cooking until the onion begins to brown. Set aside.

3. Lightly flour a work surface and roll out the dough until it is about 10 inches long. Fit it into a 3-quart baking dish with the dough going up the sides. Spoon the onion mixture into the crust, sprinkle the filling with the olives and capers, and put the cubes of cheese on the top. Fold the pointed ends in toward the center, partially enclosing the filling.

4. Bake the tart for about 40 minutes or until the crust becomes puffy and golden. Serve hot.

PER SERVING Calories: 220 • Fat: 16 g • Protein: 9 g • Sodium: 470 mg • Carbohydrates: 13 g • Fiber: 2 g

Mediterranean Stew

Serve this stew, redolent with the flavors of the sunny Mediterranean, with warmed pita bread.

INGREDIENTS | SERVES 4

3 tablespoons olive oil

3 cloves garlic, crushed and minced

1 (15½-ounce) can chickpeas, drained and rinsed

1 (19-ounce) can cannelloni beans, drained and rinsed

2 cups roasted tomatoes

1½ cups artichoke hearts, quartered

1 cup vegetable broth

4 tablespoons grated Parmesan cheese

1 teaspoon crushed red pepper, or to taste

1 teaspoon dried oregano

Salt and freshly ground black pepper, to taste

Chopped sun-dried tomatoes, for garnish

Chopped Italian parsley, for garnish

Garlic-seasoned croutons, for garnish

Crumbled feta cheese, for garnish

Fresh oregano leaves, for garnish

1. Heat the olive oil in a large saucepan over medium heat and sauté the garlic for 2–3 minutes or until golden.

2. Reduce the heat to medium low. Stir in the chickpeas, cannelloni beans, roasted tomatoes, artichoke hearts, broth, Parmesan cheese, crushed red pepper, oregano, salt, and pepper. Cook and stir for about 10 minutes. Serve in individual bowls, garnishing as desired.

PER SERVING Calories: 390 • Fat: 13 g • Protein: 15 g • Sodium: 1,180 mg • Carbohydrates: 52 g • Fiber: 9 g

Southwestern Sprouts

Don't turn up your nose at Brussels sprouts, especially when they're are kicked up a notch with seasonings and texture. You'll want to serve these often.

INGREDIENTS | SERVES 4

1 pound Brussels sprouts, trimmed and halved

1 tablespoon olive oil

1 tablespoon taco seasoning or to taste

½ cup crushed spicy taco chips

½ cup spicy or mild salsa

½ cup shredded Cheddar cheese

½ cup sunflower seeds, optional

1. Preheat the oven to 350°F.

2. Toss the sprouts with the oil and taco seasoning and put them in a roasting pan. Cook for about 30 minutes or until the sprouts become tender.

3. Put them in a serving bowl and toss with the taco chips, salsa, cheese, and sunflower seeds (if using). Serve hot.

PER SERVING Calories: 390 • Fat: 24 g • Protein: 14 g • Sodium: 680 mg • Carbohydrates: 35 g • Fiber: 8 g

Fava Bean Hummus with Pistachios

If you need extra liquid to help purée the fava beans, add olive oil or a splash of vegetable broth, but don't overdo it. The hummus should be thick, not runny. You may serve this with toasted pita pieces, bagel chips, or fresh vegetables for dunking.

INGREDIENTS | SERVES 6

1 (15-ounce) can fava beans, drained and rinsed

3 cloves garlic, or to taste

Juice from 1 lemon, or more to taste

3 tablespoons olive oil, or more as needed to process

1–2 tablespoons tahini paste

Salt and freshly ground black pepper, to taste

½ cup minced parsley

¾ cup toasted pistachios

1. Put the beans, garlic, lemon juice, olive oil, tahini, salt, and pepper into a food processor or blender and purée.

2. Spoon the mixture into a bowl and stir in the parsley and pistachios. Chill until serving time.

PER SERVING Calories: 240 • Fat: 17 g • Carbohydrates: 18 g • Protein: 8 g • Sodium: 150 mg • Fiber: 5 g

Lentil Stew

Lentils cook relatively quickly, but if you are in a hurry, use canned lentils for convenience. Offer this stew with slices of hot, buttery baguette, which you can spark with sprinkles of garlic powder, and serve with a simple salad of lightly dressed greens.

INGREDIENTS | SERVES 4

3 tablespoons olive oil

1 large sweet onion, thinly sliced

5 cloves garlic, minced

2 cups cooked lentils

3 tomatoes, quartered

2 banana peppers, stemmed and quartered lengthwise

2 Italian-style soy "sausages," thinly sliced

1 portobello mushroom, thinly sliced

½–1 cup vegetable broth, or more as needed

Salt and freshly ground black pepper, to taste

1. Heat the oil in a large skillet over medium heat and sauté the onion for 8–10 minutes or until golden. Add the garlic, lentils, tomatoes, peppers, sausages, and mushroom, stirring well.

2. Reduce the heat to medium low and continue cooking until the onions and peppers soften, about 10 minutes. Add the vegetable broth as the mixture begins to dry out. Stir in the salt and pepper. Serve hot.

PER SERVING Calories: 280 • Fat: 13 g • Protein: 12 g • Sodium: 420 mg • Carbohydrates: 31 g • Fiber: 11 g

Edamame Omelet

The addition of cheese turns this into a fusion dish.
To add more Asian flavors, stir some shredded daikon and crushed chiles to taste into the mix.

INGREDIENTS | SERVES 2

2 tablespoons olive oil

1 teaspoon minced garlic

1 bunch scallions, trimmed and cut into 1-inch pieces

½ cup shelled edamame

1 tablespoon soy sauce, or to taste

3 large eggs

½ cup shredded regular or soy Cheddar cheese

Snips of fresh cilantro, for garnish

1. Heat 2 tablespoons oil in a small skillet over medium heat and sauté the garlic and scallion for about 2 minutes. Add the edamame and soy sauce and sauté 1 minute more. Remove from the skillet and set aside.

2. Heat the remaining 1 tablespoon oil in the same skillet. Beat the eggs until mixed and pour into the hot oil. Scatter the shredded cheese on top. Lift up the edges of the omelet, tipping the skillet back and forth to cook the uncooked eggs. When the top looks firm, sprinkle the scallion mixture over half of the omelet and fold the other half over top.

3. Carefully lift the omelet out of the skillet. Divide it in half, sprinkle with the cilantro, and serve.

PER SERVING Calories: 410 • Fat: 32 g • Protein: 22 g • Sodium: 800 mg • Carbohydrates: 7 g • Fiber: 2 g

Orange Salad

A healthful salad that makes a visual impact.

INGREDIENTS | SERVES 4

3 cups cubed butternut squash, drizzled with olive oil and roasted

2 carrots, shredded

2 cups diced papaya

2 tablespoons shredded fresh ginger

Juice of 1 lime

2 tablespoons plain yogurt

1 tablespoon honey, or to taste

1 tablespoon olive oil

Salt and freshly ground black pepper, to taste

1. Combine the squash, carrots, and papaya in a large salad bowl. Set aside.

2. Stir together the ginger, lime juice, yogurt, honey, olive oil, salt, and pepper until well combined. Toss the dressing with the salad ingredients and serve.

PER SERVING Calories: 160 • Fat: 4 g • Protein: 3 g • Sodium: 40 mg • Carbohydrates: 32 g • Fiber: 7 g

Mediterranean Tofu

Because you are using silken tofu in this recipe, it will partially fall apart as you stir the dish, dispersing itself throughout the mixture.

INGREDIENTS | SERVES 4

2 tablespoons vegetable oil

1 large sweet onion, diced

4 cloves garlic, minced

3 zucchini, thinly sliced

1 (14½-ounce) can crushed tomatoes

1 (1 pound) package silken firm tofu, cubed

1 cup pitted kalamata olives

1. Heat the oil in a large wok or skillet and sauté the onion and garlic for about 3 minutes.

2. Add the zucchini and cook 3 minutes more.

3. Add the tomatoes, tofu, and olives and cook 2–3 minutes more. Serve.

PER SERVING Calories: 290 • Fat: 18 g • Protein: 12 g • Sodium: 650 mg • Carbohydrates: 23 g • Fiber: 5 g

CHAPTER 15

Special Nutritional Concerns

Nutritional concerns are causing more and more people to seek nutritional advice. However, the plethora of advice available from many sources can seem overwhelming and sometimes misdirected. Many concerns are individualized, because we are not all built the same way. Different foods can affect two people in different ways, even if they have the same diagnosis. Therefore, the best thing you can do is listen to your system—it will send messages to you if you let it. This chapter will guide you in dealing with special nutritional concerns. Other tools and support from a doctor, registered dietitian, journaling, and counseling can be extremely helpful as well.

Eating Disorders

The teen years can be difficult for both boys and girls. Looks are extremely important for most teens, who focus mainly on body image. Often teens have unrealistic notions about the way their bodies should look. Boys usually put more emphasis on exercising, especially with weights. Teenage girls tend to diet as they strive for the perfect body. This usually involves some type of fad diet, and that can be very dangerous, especially during the adolescent years. Concerns about weight can also lead girls to engage in unhealthy behaviors, such as excessive exercise, self-induced vomiting, and the abuse of medications such as laxatives or diuretics.

Being obsessive about weight can result in various eating disorders. An estimated one million or more Americans suffer from some type of eating disorder. Eating disorders are more than a food problem and are linked to psychological problems.

Anorexia and Bulimia

Anorexia nervosa is a common eating disorder that usually begins at the age of fourteen or fifteen (but can occur at a younger age), with another peak in incidence among eighteen-year-olds. It is more common in adolescent girls, but is also found in boys and its incidence has been increasing. Anorexia causes an overwhelming fear of being overweight and a drive to be thin, leading to self-induced starvation or an extreme restriction of calories that can lead to being severely underweight. Anorexia is linked to menstrual irregularity, osteoporosis (brittle bone disease) in women, and a greater risk of early death in both men and women.

Bulimia, another eating disorder, is marked by a loss of control and binge eating, followed by purging behaviors. The person gorges on high-calorie foods and then intentionally vomits or uses laxatives or diuretics.

Signs to Watch For

If you suspect that your child has an eating disorder, here are some factors to look for:

- Low self-esteem
- Recent weight loss of 15 percent or more of normal body weight, with no medical reason
- A fear of gaining weight or of being overweight
- Purging behaviors (vomiting or using diuretics—water pills—or laxatives to lose weight)
- Having a distorted image of body size or shape (for example, believing she is overweight even though she is at a healthy weight or even underweight)
- A preoccupation with thoughts of food, calories, and weight
- Restrictive eating patterns such as frequently skipping meals, fasting, or eliminating entire food groups
- A preference for eating alone
- For young women, amenorrhea (absence of menstrual cycles) or delayed onset of puberty
- Being underweight, with a body mass index that is below normal
- Exercising compulsively
- An extreme denial of the possibility of eating disorder
- Withdrawal from friends and family
- Wearing bulky clothing to hide weight loss
- A recent or past event in life that was very stressful

You should have your child seen by a physician as soon as possible if you think she or he might have an eating disorder. Eating disorders can cause extreme undernourishment and even death. The best treatment for eating disorders combines medical, psychological, and nutrition counseling.

ESSENTIAL

For more information about eating disorders, contact the National Eating Disorders Association at *www.nationaleatingdisorders.org* or the Renfrew Center at *www.renfrew.org*.

Religious Restrictions

Many religions include dietary laws. Jewish and Muslim dietary laws are similar, one following the Law of Moses, the other keeping in step with the notion of clean and unclean. Hindus and Buddhists are mainly vegetarian, although meat and fish are allowed following strict guidelines. Early Christian food rules banned the consumption of meat offered to idols, blood, and things that were strangled. Roman Catholics abstained from meat on Fridays until the Second Vatican Council (Vatican II) amended the laws in the 1960s.

Kosher Foods

Kosher is the English word for kashrut, or the Hebrew dietary laws derived from the Torah's book of Leviticus. Foods that are not kosher are treif. The only animals that may be eaten are those deemed clean, which include quadrupeds that chew their cud and have completely split hooves, fish with both fins and scales, domesticated birds, locusts, and grasshoppers.

Kosher slaughter and preparation of food is strictly regulated. Animals must be killed in a clean and humane manner to limit the animal's suffering and demonstrate the responsibility that comes with having power over life and death. In preparing meat, body fat and sinuous tendons must be removed, and the body must be drained completely of all fluids.

Specific food combinations are prohibited. An animal may not be seethed (boiled) in its mother's milk. This act is seen as a symbolic combination of life and death and is interpreted in modern times as the prohibition of meat and milk in any form being cooked or eaten together. This includes placing food in the same dish or eating this combination at the same meal. Fish and meat are also not to be consumed together, and certain holidays require that specific foods be eaten.

FACT

Following kosher law is an act of faith, although many scholars continue to explore the health benefits of the kosher diet. It appears to be a more hygienic, less toxic diet overall.

Kosher foods in the market are marked with a symbol that indicates they have been certified by a rabbi or rabbinical authority. Symbols include a U, OU, and K. In addition, foods containing specific ingredients are clearly labeled, including D for dairy, P for fish, M for meat, and Pareve, which means no meat or dairy products.

Fad Diets

The billion-dollar industry shows the demand for fad dieting is increasing. Today, millions of people are dieting to aid weight loss, weight gain, or meet a particular nutritional need. The food and nutrition industry has become more focused on marketing and being able to meet the short-term dieting demand. Americans seem to be moving further away from basic nutrition and closer to quick fixes and easy answers touted by fad diets. The abundance of nutrition information on food labels, in new studies, on television, and on the Internet may actually be creating more confusion. As a result, people may throw up their hands and turn to fad diets that appeal to them. The problem is, fad diets are temporary plans that make false promises. It's better to develop an individual diet focused on foods that are right for your own body, which will become a lifetime plan for overall health.

No single dietary regimen works for everyone, which is why so many different approaches exist. It is important to understand the facts of any diet before jumping into a "too good to be true" plan. For example, some programs emphasize "rapid weight loss." However, you have to be extremely careful not to lose muscle, bone, and water with this sometimes dangerous approach. Most people who lose weight this way end up regaining more pounds after they finish the diet than they lost.

Balance is the desired outcome in an overall health plan, but balance is often absent in fad diets. These programs tend to be very strict, with limited food choices and complicated lists of what not to eat. Diets, such as cabbage soup and grapefruit, focus on monotonous food choices. Obviously, several food groups are absent, including some that supply the body's main sources of energy. Not only are you likely to get bored undertaking one of these diets, you could miss out on critical nutrients and develop negative relationships with certain important foods.

Many people try numerous diets before they are truly ready to build a new, healthier lifestyle. Fad diets might start you thinking about taking action. They can increase your readiness to make changes. They can be tools, but they are not fixes. They can be used as a starting point, but only your ability to follow through with long-term changes will produce lasting, healthy results.

A diet is the food you eat for a lifetime. Dietary habits can change depending on your health and beliefs. The best approach for achieving long-term success is to move slow and steady. Determine where you want to go, then develop a series of steps to work on one at a time to create a solid base that supports behavior changes. Each goal you set will include certain steps and skills to practice. Fad diets could prevent the development of real skills. So, although a fad diet may sound tempting, ask yourself if it will help you change your relationships with food. Getting back to basics is a better way to achieve your goals for weight loss and overall health.

Top reasons not to go fad:

- No specific food melts fat.
- It isn't healthy to unnaturally speed up your metabolism using a product made in a factory or lab.
- Avoiding an entire food group won't produce benefits, just imbalances in your body.
- Weight loss relies on effort, not miracles.

Visit *www.EatRight.org* to read up-to-date reviews on today's diets. Here are some of the more popular ones:

- **5 Factor Diet.** This plan introduces many beneficial behaviors to promote weight loss with a nutritionally balanced diet. However, it is presented as a 5-week plan instead of a long-term lifestyle to promote weight loss and weight management.
- **Aktins.** It is never a good idea to decrease the amount of vegetables and fruits you consume, especially if you're trying to prevent cancer and other chronic illnesses. It's impossible to generate rapid weight loss and sustain it without eating fruits and vegetables, which provide

low-caloric density. You're likely to burn out and regain the weight you lost just as quickly.

- **Cabbage Soup Diet.** This diet lacks adequate amounts of protein and other macronutrients and micronutrients, putting you at risk for losing lean body mass. It is basically a fast, which can promote weight loss, but you'll probably regain that weight shortly after completing the diet.

- **Grapefruit Diet.** Any diet that eliminates whole food groups is creating an unbalanced eating environment and putting you at risk for losing lean body mass. This is not healthy for your body composition, immune system, or bone health.

- **South Beach Diet.** Most phases of this diet are well balanced. However, it is another short-term plan. The restrictive phase could also cause you to burn out before you even start the other phases.

- **The 4 Day Diet.** This is a very restrictive diet that does not encourage you to create a positive long-term relationship with food. It is too low in calories on some days. It also provides inadequate amounts of carbohydrates and some key nutrients, such as vitamin D and calcium.

- **The Belly Fat Cure.** This diet may put you at risk for vitamin and mineral deficiencies, because it limits the amount of fruit and dairy products you consume, due to Cruise's claim that natural sugar contributes to belly fat. Some menus provided seem to be low in fiber and calcium and high in sodium and cholesterol.

- **The Raw Food Diet.** Although this diet includes many nutrient-dense foods, it may be very difficult for many people to achieve. It is also extremely hard to ensure you are getting adequate nutrition and preventing vitamin deficiencies with this diet.

Diabetes

The American Diabetic Association estimates that 18 million Americans suffer from diabetes. Diabetes is a disease in which the body does not produce or adequately utilize insulin. Insulin is a hormone made in the pancreas; it is needed to convert sugar, starches, and other food into energy. People with diabetes have trouble controlling their blood sugar levels because their bodies do not properly produce or use insulin. As a result, blood sugar, or glucose, accumulates in the blood and makes blood sugar levels rise. Instead of being used for energy as it should be, sugar passes out of the body through the urine. This puts an extra strain on the kidneys, causing frequent urination and excessive thirst. The cause of diabetes is a mystery, although genetic and environmental factors such as obesity and lack of exercise seem to play definite roles.

Types of Diabetes

There are three types of diabetes. In Type 1 diabetes, the pancreas produces no insulin. This type can affect anyone, but occurs most often in children and young adults, accounting for only about 5 to 10 percent of diabetes cases. Its main cause is genetic. Type 1 diabetics must take daily insulin injections to survive.

Type 2 diabetes is a metabolic disorder in which the body does not properly make or use insulin. It is the most common form of diabetes, affecting 90 to 95 percent of people with the disease. Being overweight or obese is a common risk factor for this type of diabetes. It can usually be controlled through diet and exercise. Type 2 diabetes is nearing epidemic proportions, due to an increased number of older Americans and a greater prevalence of obesity and sedentary lifestyles.

Type 3 diabetes is gestational diabetes, which can occur during pregnancy. It is usually the result of changing hormones within a woman's body. It needs to be carefully controlled throughout the pregnancy and usually disappears once the baby is born. Women who have gestational diabetes are at a higher risk of developing it in later pregnancies.

ALERT

Uncontrolled diabetes can cause major health problems and can even be life threatening. It is a major risk factor for heart disease, poor circulation, eye disorders, foot problems, and kidney disorders. In addition to taking your diabetes medication or insulin as instructed by your doctor, you can influence your blood sugar and your health in a positive way by improving your diet, exercising, and reducing your stress levels.

Celiac Disease

Celiac disease is a food-related condition that is often lifelong. It is also known as gluten intolerance, nontropical sprue, or gluten-sensitive enteropathy. This condition can occur at any age and is much more common than once thought. Celiac disease is an intestinal disorder in which gluten, a natural protein commonly found in many grains including wheat, barley, rye, and oats, cannot be tolerated by the body.

When gluten is metabolized in the body, it breaks down into glutenin and gliadin; it is the gliadin that does the damage. When people with celiac disease consume foods with gluten or gliadin, the immune system responds by damaging the villi or the walls of the small intestines that help to absorb nutrients. The intestine cannot absorb nutrients properly, and the person can become malnourished. Celiac disease is known as an autoimmune disease because the immune system is actually causing the damage.

Symptoms

Celiac disease can affect people differently, and symptoms and severity can vary. Some common symptoms include:

- Chronic diarrhea that does not get better with medication
- Foul-smelling, greasy, pale stools
- Gassiness
- Recurring abdominal bloating
- Weight loss
- Fatigue
- Infertility, lack of menstruation
- Bone or joint pain
- Depression, irritability, or mood changes
- Neurological problems, including weakness, poor balance, seizures, headaches, or numbness or tingling in the legs
- Itchy, painful skin rash
- Tooth discoloration or loss of enamel, sores on lips or tongue
- Other signs of vitamin deficiency, such as scaly skin or hyperkeratosis (from lack of vitamin A), or bleeding gums or bruising easily (from lack of vitamin K)

Treatment

Celiac disease is a genetic disorder, so there is nothing you can do to prevent it. A person with the disorder must follow a gluten-restricted, gliadin-free diet for life in order to successfully manage the condition. Once gliadin is eliminated from the diet, the small intestines can begin to heal, nutrient absorption will improve, and symptoms will begin to disappear.

To eliminate gliadin from the diet, any foods or food components with the following four grains must be completely eliminated: wheat, rye, barley, and oats. Avoiding wheat can be a very big dietary challenge because wheat is the main ingredient in so many different foods.

To help deal with gluten intolerance, follow some of these guidelines:

- Consult a registered dietitian for information, education, and help on eating a gliadin-free diet.
- Look for gluten-free grains and other food products at specialty stores or on the Internet.
- Read food labels carefully, and become familiar with the lingo that can indicate the presence of gliadin. A dietitian can help you with this.
- Become educated about the origin and composition of ingredients. For example, vinegar may seem harmless, but it is often distilled from a grain with gliadin and would not be appropriate if you have gluten intolerance. Choose rice vinegar, wine vinegar, or pure cider vinegar instead.
- Use gliadin-free flour in place of wheat or white flour when cooking or baking. These types of flours include corn, rice, soy, arrowroot, tapioca, and potato flours. They are a bit different than wheat flour, so it may take some experimentation.
- When eating away from home, make sure to ask questions when necessary or pack your own gluten-free foods when traveling.
- Contact food manufacturers for current information on their ingredient lists. These are constantly changing, so you need to stay up-to-date.
- Seek out local and national support groups. These groups can be a great way to share information with people with your condition. A registered dietitian or the Internet can help you find these groups.

According to the National Institutes of Health, an estimated 1 in 4,700 Americans have been diagnosed with celiac disease. However, it may be much more common than this. Celiac disease is the most common genetic disease in Europe.

It is vital to know the difference between gluten and gliadin when checking food labels or asking for ingredient information from manufacturers. These terms may indicate that a food contains gliadin:

- Flour, self-rising flour, enriched flour
- Malt or cereal extracts
- Malt flavoring
- Modified food starch
- Distilled vinegar
- Monosodium glutamate (MSG)
- Emulsifiers
- Hydrolyzed vegetable protein (HVP)
- Stabilizers
- Cereals
- Wheat starch

Keep in mind that the information given in this section only skims the surface of what you need to know to manage this condition. Seek the help of a doctor and dietitian to receive all the information you need. If you think you may have gluten intolerance, do not self-diagnose. Consult your doctor immediately.

Lactose Intolerance

Don't confuse lactose intolerance with a milk allergy. Being lactose intolerant means you have an intolerance to the sugar in milk (lactose) because your body does not produce enough of the enzyme lactase, which is responsible for the digestion of lactose. Left undigested, lactose can cause uncomfortable symptoms such as nausea, cramping, bloating, abdominal pain, gas, and diarrhea.

ALERT

People who have a true milk allergy are allergic to the protein found in milk, and they must avoid all milk products.

Lactose intolerance can affect people in varying degrees. Some have severe symptoms when they ingest lactose, whereas others can consume some lactose. Symptoms can begin anywhere from fifteen minutes to several hours after consuming food or a drink containing lactose. To help deal with lactose intolerance, follow some of these basic guidelines:

- Look for label ingredient terms that suggest lactose is present, such as milk, dry milk solids, nonfat milk solids, buttermilk, lactose, malted milk, sour or sweet cream, margarine, milk chocolate, whey, whey protein concentrate, and cheese.
- If your intolerance is severe, it is vital to recognize baked and processed food products that might contain lactose, such as pancakes, biscuits, cookies, cakes, salad dressings, commercial sauces or gravies, cream soups, lunchmeats, whipped toppings, and powdered coffee creamers.
- Look for lactose-reduced or lactose-free milk products.
- Experiment so you know what you can tolerate. Start with small amounts, and then gradually increase the portion size to determine your personal tolerance level.
- Consume lactose-containing foods as part of a meal instead of alone. This can sometimes make the lactose easier to digest.
- Eat smaller portions of lactose-containing foods. For example, instead of drinking a whole glass of milk, just try half of a serving.
- Choose calcium-rich foods that are naturally low in lactose; aged cheeses such as Swiss, Colby, Parmesan, and Cheddar are good choices.
- Try eating yogurt. Many people who are lactose intolerant can tolerate yogurt because of its "friendly" bacteria, which help digest the lactose.

- Don't forget about other calcium-rich nondairy foods, including dark green leafy vegetables, calcium-fortified orange juice, and canned sardines or salmon with bones.
- Look for kosher foods that have the words "parev" or "parve" on the label. This means they are milk-free.

If you suspect you may have lactose intolerance, do not self-diagnose. This condition can be linked to other health issues.

CHAPTER 16

Food Allergies

Food allergies are an immune-system reaction to protein molecules found in food. This reaction is actually a mistake your body makes. Your immune system is set up to defend your body against viruses, toxins, and bacteria—foreign invaders that have no place in the body. When cells in your body think of food as a foreign invader they attack, producing the reactions known as symptoms of an allergy. In the case of a true food allergy, reaction time is usually within minutes to two hours.

What Is a Food Allergy?

You cannot be allergic to a substance your body hasn't been exposed to. Therefore, you won't have a reaction the first time you eat a food your body decides to attack. This is called sensitizing. No one knows why this overre-action occurs. Scientists are studying various theories, but no one has an answer yet.

Allergens and Antigens

When the protein, also called an antigen, of the allergenic food meets some of the cells in your body, the cells produce an antibody specifically created to bind to the antigen in the food. These antibodies, also known as Immunoglobulin E (IgE), attach themselves to large cells called mast cells and basophils, forming a complex that is now ready to defend your body.

The next time you come in contact with that food antigen, it fits into the antibody like a key into a lock, releasing chemicals from the mast cells that provoke your body into a response. Those chemicals include histamines, which cause swelling of tissue, itching, hives, breathing problems, and irregular heartbeat. Food allergy symptoms include:

- Itching
- Hives
- Eczema
- Swelling of the lips, tongue, and mouth
- Breathing difficulties
- Coughing
- Stuffy nose and congestion
- Gastrointestinal (GI) problems (vomiting, diarrhea)
- Irregular heartbeat
- Anaphylaxis

TH1 and TH2 Cells

Your immune system has two main branches of white blood cells that respond to real and perceived threats to the body. One is called TH1, which is responsible for corralling and neutralizing bacteria and viruses. The other is called TH2, which reacts to substances such as protein molecules in food.

I never had allergies as a child; why am I allergic now?
You can develop allergies to any substance at any time of your life. Scientists aren't sure why these allergies develop. Anytime you experience any of the symptoms in the allergy-symptom list, get to a doctor or emergency room quickly for medications that may help prevent a life-threatening reaction.

These two branches are joined by regulatory cells that track, monitor, and regulate the TH1 and TH2 cells. It may be that if your immune system isn't stimulated by bacteria and viruses at an early age, the regulatory or helper cells don't learn how to control the TH1 and TH2 cells, and they will overreact. Autoimmune diseases such as celiac disease and multiple sclerosis can result from overactive TH1 cells. Food allergies result from overactive TH2 cells.

The Diagnosis

There are several ways to diagnose a food allergy, including medical tests, food challenges, elimination diets, and self-screening. Mild allergies can be difficult to diagnose, but if your reaction has been severe, the suspect food can usually be quickly identified.

Start with Yourself

A self-screening test can be helpful, and is usually the first step toward an accurate diagnosis. Start keeping a food diary, and carefully observe and record your symptoms: when symptoms occur; which foods you have eaten and how much you consumed; time from eating the food to when symptoms appeared; and the severity of symptoms.

Visit the Doctor

Most people visit their doctors when they are not feeling well. You may have had digestive problems, skin irritations, breathing problems, depression, or fatique and weakness. Your doctor will do a general workup on you, and if you are in general good health, the sleuthing begins.

When you begin the journey to diagnosis, find an allergy specialist. General practitioners and internists do not have the experience in diagnostic tools and treatments that specialists do. General practitioners can do preliminary work and exclude some diseases, but when interpreting test results, a specialist is more qualified. The following organizations can help you find a qualified specialist:

- American Academy of Allergy, Asthma and Immunology
- American Board of Medical Specialists
- American College of Allergy, Asthma and Immunology
- American Board of Allergy and Immunology
- National Institute of Allergy and Infectious Diseases

Get Tested

Two basic types of medical tests are used to diagnose allergies: skin tests and RAST (radioallergosorbent test). The RAST is a blood test that looks for the presence of IgEs specific to different foods. Your IgE number must be above a certain threshold for diagnosis of a food allergy.

The skin-prick test, while less accurate than the RAST, is also less expensive and faster. A solution containing the suspect proteins is scratched onto the skin, along with a control of salt water. The size of the reaction determines the allergy, with a negative reaction being the most accurate diagnosis. After a statistically significant positive skin test, the RAST test is the next step.

For the RAST (also called CAP-RAST and ImmunoCap test), blood is drawn and tested against the different antigens from the suspect food. If IgEs are found with numbers above a certain threshold, a diagnosis of a food allergy is made. The higher the score, the more accurate the diagnosis. Doctors have set thresholds (in kUA/L, or kilounits of antibody per liter) above which there is a 95 percent chance that you do have an allergy to that food.

▼ **95 Percent Diagnostic Certainty CAP-RAST Test (0 to 100)**

Allergen	kUA/L Number
Peanuts	14
Wheat	80
Eggs	7
Milk	15
Fish	20
Shellfish	20
Soy	65
Tree nuts	15

Other Tests

The elimination diet is a less scientific, but simple, way of determining food allergies when medical tests are inconclusive or contradictory. With this diet, which should be planned with the help of a nutritionist to make sure the diet is wholesome and meets all your needs, you start on some hypoallergenic foods, including rice, bananas, vegetables, millet, and lamb.

Once you start feeling better, other foods are added slowly, at the rate of one every few days to a week. This is called the challenge phase of the diagnosis. If symptoms appear, the suspect food can be identified. Keeping a food diary is critical during this test. If allergy reactions have been life threatening, this test should only be conducted in a physician's office where appropriate remedies are available.

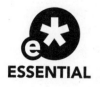

ESSENTIAL

You may see ads or pamphlets for other types of allergy tests that are not accepted by the medical community. Don't waste your time and money on hair testing, NAET, energy pathway diagnosis, kinesiology, cytotoxic food testing, the IgG ELISA test, Vega, or electrodermal testing. These tests have not been peer reviewed using double-blind studies and are unproven.

The rotation diet is another possible diagnostic tool. For some people with less severe allergies, the rotation diet may prevent future allergies. It can also uncover allergies to other foods, including corn, tomatoes, strawberries, and yeast. In the rotation system, a very strict diet of only a certain number of biologically related foods is eaten every day for four or five days.

The premise is that "masking antibodies" your body produces for a food will diminish in that time frame, because your immune system "rests" when not exposed to those allergens. This diet should not be followed long-term because it limits entire food groups necessary for good health. Some doctors think this diet does not work. It is very limiting and can be quite challenging to maintain. Although the diet may be a diagnostic tool, claims that it can cure food allergies should be viewed with skepticism. Only you and your doctor can decide if a rotation diet is a good tool for you.

Now What?

Once you have a firm diagnosis, it's time to start learning which foods you must avoid and how to prepare for any potential reactions. Your doctor may prescribe an emergency kit including oral antihistamines along with an Epi-Pen, which is a small syringe filled with epinephrine. It's important that you review the instructions with this kit, and even stage a mock emergency so you understand how to use the kit and can implement the medication as quickly as possible. If your child is allergic, inform all the key people in his life about the allergy, so they can eliminate these foods and watch for symptoms of a reaction.

ALERT

You may have heard of food challenges or oral challenges, where you are fed increasing amounts of the suspect food to see when a reaction occurs. Never attempt this outside of a doctor's office. A doctor and lifesaving equipment must be on hand. Although this test can lead to an accurate diagnosis, it also carries a high risk. To get an accurate result, you must not be taking antihistamines.

Not only should you educate yourself and your family about your allergy, educate the community you live in as well. Wear a medical-alert bracelet, let those close to you (teachers, friends) know about the allergy, and keep an emergency kit on hand to deal with the allergies.

Ask your doctor for a list of words and terms that cover your food allergy, and bring it with you when you shop and when you eat in restaurants. Become familiar with these terms so you know what to look for when reading food labels.

Why Are Cases Increasing?

Food allergy rates around the world are skyrocketing. Twenty years ago, perhaps one or two children in an entire school population had a severe allergy; today there are at least ten times as many. What is causing this increase?

Genetics

Scientists believe many, if not most, food allergies have a genetic basis. That is, if food allergies run in your family, your chances of developing one are increased. If both parents have food allergies, there is a 60 percent chance that at least one of their children will have an allergy. But even if there is no history of food allergies in the family, 5–15 percent of children will develop one.

Too Clean, or Too Dirty

You may have heard warnings about overuse of antibiotics and antibacterial cleansers. Not only do these practices force bacteria and viruses to mutate, but the evolved germs can become resistant to current drugs and medicines. And there's another angle: Children who grow up in a very clean environment don't develop as many antibodies to germs, so their immune systems may be underused or "bored" and will strike out against other substances, such as food. This is called the Hygiene Hypothesis.

Studies have shown that allergies are less common in children who attend day care and early preschool; who grow up in rural areas, especially farms; who have pets; and who have older brothers and sisters who bring germs and illnesses home from school.

Conversely, inner-city children, children of smokers, and children who live in very polluted areas have more allergies and food sensitivities. Rates of asthma are particularly high in the most polluted areas. Therefore, environmental toxins and pollution may play a role in allergy development.

Should I ditch the soap?
Proponents of the Hygiene Hypothesis don't want you to stop washing your hands or cleaning the kitchen. But using plain soap and water instead of antibacterial solutions and soaps may lead to a healthier family. Children who play in the dirt, have pets, and contract normal childhood diseases can be healthier than those who are overly protected.

Moderation May Be Key

The lesson may be to simply avoid the extremes. Don't become obsessed with cleanliness. Let your children play in the dirt and with animals, and don't shy away from everyone who sneezes.

Finally, don't smoke! Smoking is a proven cause of a wide range of maladies, including asthma, SIDS, allergies, bronchitis, and cancer. Secondhand smoke is particularly dangerous for children.

Eight Allergenic Foods

Eight foods comprise 90 percent of all food allergies. They are peanuts, tree nuts, wheat, milk, eggs, soy, shellfish, and fish. A person may be allergic to just one of these foods, or may have multiple allergies to two or more of these substances.

Peanuts

An allergy to peanuts is the most publicized and widely known because news reports have pointed out spectacular anaphylactic reactions to unbelievably minute quantities of the peanut protein. There are a few reasons why peanut allergies can be so severe.

The protein responsible for the allergy has a unique shape that is very easy for your immune system to recognize. All proteins have bends and folds in their structures, but the peanut proteins are folded so the allergenic molecules are right on the surface.

QUESTION

Is it aflatoxin?
Recently, a company made a claim that their product, which contains peanuts, is safe for people who are allergic to peanuts because the peanuts did not have aflatoxin, a mold that can grow on the nut. This is a misleading and dangerous claim, because peanut allergies have nothing to do with mold. It's the protein in peanuts that causes the reaction.

Three specific protein molecules in peanuts, called Ara h 1, 2, and 3, provoke an allergic reaction. Your immune system has three times the targets and three times the potential response with peanuts compared to other foods that generate allergic reactions. The antibody in your blood that is created when you have a peanut allergy is called PN-IgE.

Milk

Two main types of milk allergies exist: slow onset and rapid onset. Rapid onset can occur within minutes of consuming the milk protein. Symptoms include itching, hives, difficulty breathing, and anaphylaxis. It is less common than slow onset, which is manifested in vomiting, fussiness in babies, and failure to thrive. The slow-onset allergy can be more difficult to diagnose, as the RAST test isn't very accurate for this type.

Most milk allergies are reactions to both the casein and whey portions of the milk protein. The casein protein is heat stable, that is, cooking will not destroy its configuration. Heated milk products are therefore still allergenic. Whey is not heat stable, so if your allergy is to the protein in whey only, you may be able to consume heated milk products.

FACT

Food intolerance is not the same as food allergy. Food intolerance is a reaction to a food, food additives, and food colorings, which takes place solely in the digestive tract. The immune system is not involved in food intolerance. One of the most common food intolerances is lactose intolerance: a reaction to lactase, the sugar found in milk.

When you're looking for milk or cheese substitutes, it can help to look for the word "vegan." Vegan means that no animal products whatsoever were used in making that food. The word "pareve" can also be a good clue. This is a kosher term meaning no dairy or meat.

The good news about milk allergies is that most children outgrow them after avoiding milk and milk products for one to two years. However, if a young child is allergic to milk, the odds are fairly good that she will develop allergies to other foods as well.

Fish and Shellfish

There is usually no cross-reactivity to shellfish (shrimp, crab, and lobster) and finfish (grouper, haddock, walleye), but some people are allergic to both. If you have a severe allergy to one or the other, it's best to simply avoid both.

This allergy can, and does, occur at any time of life, not only in childhood. It's a tricky allergy to manage because of cross-contamination. Cross-contamination in this subgroup can occur when the oil used to fry shrimp is then used to cook French fries. Or a spoon that contained fish-based Worcestershire sauce could contaminate a salad.

ESSENTIAL

Some people who have a fish allergy can actually consume certain species of fish. The canning process that tuna and salmon undergo may remove the allergenic proteins. Also, some people allergic to shellfish (shrimp) aren't always allergic to mollusks (clams, oysters). An elimination diet or food challenge, only in your doctor's presence, will help determine the extent of your allergy.

Fish proteins can even become airborne during the cooking process and can cause reactions. Make sure the fish you do eat is very fresh. Fish that has begun to spoil will have a buildup of histamine in the flesh, which can cause a reaction even in people who are not allergic. Iodine is not the cause of fish allergies, as many people believe; the reaction is to the protein in fish.

Eggs

The proteins in egg whites cause most of the allergic reactions in people who are allergic to eggs. Uncooked or poorly cooked egg whites can cause the most severe reactions. But some people are also allergic to the proteins in egg yolks. This is another one of the very serious reactions that can be life threatening. Some people who are allergic to eggs can even get a reaction from skin contact with egg products or from inhaling fumes from cooking eggs.

One of the best ways to avoid eggs is to read labels. With the new labeling requirements now in effect, look for terms such as "made in a facility that also processes eggs." But, as with all processed foods, mistakes can happen. It's a good idea to become familiar with the names eggs can hide behind in processed foods, and scan the ingredient list even if the label reassures you the product doesn't contain egg. Again, the word "vegan" is probably your best clue, because these foods are made with no animal products whatsoever.

People generally outgrow egg allergies. Most allergies begin in young children, who outgrow the reaction by age five. Food challenges are usually used to diagnose egg allergies.

Some vaccines, including the flu vaccine and the shot for measles/mumps/rubella, are developed and made using egg proteins. Your doctor can actually test the vaccine to see if it contains egg proteins before it is administered to you or your child.

Wheat

An allergy to wheat is sometimes a reaction to the gluten, or protein, found in wheat and some other grains; other times it's a reaction to the grain itself. A pure reaction to wheat is different from celiac disease, also known as celiac sprue. Some researchers think gluten allergies may go far beyond celiac disease, and if there are IgE antibodies to gluten in the blood, avoiding gluten may improve symptoms.

If you are allergic to wheat, you may also want to avoid barley, rye, triticale, and perhaps oats. Cross-contamination can be a problem with wheat allergies, so make sure the grains you consume are pure, from the field to the packing plant.

Starting in 2008, the Food and Drug Administration tightened guidelines for food labeling. Standards apply to products labeled "gluten free," which help people who are allergic to gluten more readily identify safe foods. Guidelines labeling other allergenic foods were put into effect in January 2006. However, there is a caveat with this rule. The claim "gluten free" will only apply to products containing wheat. Oats, barley, rye, and triticale, which can be sources of gluten through cross-contamination, are not included in this claim, so you still must read labels carefully.

Gluten can hide in lots of foods that seem innocuous. Thoroughly study labels on all the processed foods you buy and learn about these hidden sources. The only way to be safe is to examine labels on all foods more complicated than lettuce. Gluten can be found in some unlikely places including:

- Sour cream, ice cream, and cheese
- Nondairy creamers
- Meat patties and sausages
- Soy meat substitutes
- Malt flavoring and caramel coloring
- Rice mixes and seasoning mixes
- Some medications
- Canned soups and bouillon cubes
- Salad dressing, mustard, flavored vinegars, and mayonnaise
- Canned baked beans and vegetables with sauces
- Nonstick baking sprays with flour
- Cocoa mixes and chocolate drinks

Wheat allergies can be difficult to diagnose because skin tests and blood tests are usually inconclusive. An elimination diet, under the supervision of a doctor or nutritionist, may be your best bet.

Soy

Soy is a legume, as are peanuts. If you are allergic to peanuts, you may have a cross-reactivity to soy or other legumes, including chickpeas, lima beans, and Great Northern beans. But an allergy to one does not guarantee an allergy to another.

It's rare for adults to develop an allergy to soy. Soy allergies usually develop at around three months, and many children outgrow it. The allergy usually begins as a reaction to soy-based formulas; breastfeeding is one of the best ways to prevent allergies to soy and milk.

ALERT

Soy can hide behind certain terms in food that aren't included in labeling laws. "Vegetable protein" and "natural flavors" are blanket terms manufacturers are allowed to use for products that can contain soy. Monoglycerides and diglycerides may be derived from soy, so avoid foods that include those terms on the label.

Some of the symptoms more unique to soy allergies include skin reactions such as eczema and acne, along with canker sores and hives. These reactions are more uncomfortable than life threatening, although an anaphylactic reaction is still possible. For mild reactions, taking an antihistamine will help reduce symptoms.

You have five different types of taste buds on your tongue: sweet, salty, sour, bitter, and umami. Umami is less commonly known and understood. In 2000, researchers isolated the receptor for umami and officially added it to the types of taste buds. It is a "meaty" taste triggered by the presence of glutamate amino acids, found in soy sauce, mushrooms, and monosodium glutamate.

If you are allergic to soy, you must omit soy sauce from your diet, or use a substitute you make at home. You'll have to carefully read labels of medications, too. Some of the fast-melt medicines are soy-based.

Tree Nuts

As with peanut allergies, tree-nut allergies can be very severe and usually last your entire life. If you have an allergy to peanuts, there is about a 40–50 percent chance you will develop an allergy to tree nuts as well. Nuts can hide in processed and prepared foods, and cross-contamination is a great risk, even if the food has been properly labeled. Avoid all nut butters and pastes as well. Tree nuts include:

- Walnuts
- Pecans
- Pistachios
- Chestnuts
- Hazelnuts
- Almonds
- Macadamia nuts
- Cashews
- Beechnuts
- Brazil nuts

Nut oils may or may not be safe for you to eat. The processing that extracts oil from nuts usually removes the allergenic proteins. But if you have a severe allergy, it's best to simply avoid all nut oils. Natural extracts such as almond extract should also be avoided. Also be aware that nut products and oils can be found in some lotions and shampoos; skin contact can trigger a severe reaction in people with these allergies.

Coconut, water chestnuts, and nutmeg are not part of the tree-nut family. Unless you are specifically allergic to these foods, they don't cross-react with the tree-nut families.

Cross-Contamination

One of the most insidious problems for people with food allergies and celiac disease is cross-contamination. From buying a food from a factory that uses peanuts to eating oatmeal grown in a field next to a wheat field, cross-contamination is a serious health risk. But you can take steps to minimize this risk.

Dedicated Mill

When you buy soy, potato, millet, or any other type of gluten-free flour, look for the words "dedicated mill" on the label. This means that the mill only produces that particular kind of flour, so there is less chance of cross-contamination with gluten. If your allergies are severe, you may even want to find a company that purchases raw produce from farms that do not rotate their crops.

The same is true for peanut and nut allergies. If a nut-free candy is made in the same building as one that has nuts, cross-contamination becomes a real issue. Look for products from companies that guarantee nut-free manufacturing environments. Be on the lookout for recalls, too; mistakes do happen.

Clean Kitchens

If you have a severe allergy, the foods you eat must come from clean kitchens. This doesn't mean bacteria free, but it means free of cross-contamination. In restaurants, oil that was used to fry fish can contaminate the potatoes that are fried next.

In the case of peanuts, more than any other food, allergic reactions to an incredibly tiny amount of the protein can be spectacular and very serious. Cross-contamination can be caused by using the same spatula to transfer peanut cookies and sugar cookies to a cooling rack. Concentrations as low as 1 in 10,000 can trigger the immune response.

The Plan

Once you have been diagnosed and understand how to manage your allergy, you should develop a plan. Clean out your pantry, removing all suspect foods. Collect recipes that omit your allergens. Get used to reading labels. Keep your allergy kit with you at all times. Aggressively ask questions of people who serve you food.

How to Read Labels

In January 2006, the FDA changed standards on food labels to make it easier to find suspect foods in the products you buy. The product must clearly state if it contains any of the eight groups of foods most responsible for allergic reactions. The language is simple: If a product contains casein, a milk protein, the label has to show the words "contains milk," or if it has some seitan, the label must read "contains gluten."

FACT

Genetic engineering may be a future solution to food allergies. Scientists have been able to produce hypoallergenic strains of food-allergy molecules that can be used in treatments. The treatments could also have few, if any, side effects. These treatments may be some years in the future, but the research is promising.

A few words of warning: the word "free" isn't regulated by the FDA. A product that says "milk free" may still contain milk protein. And the phrase "may contain" can be a blanket legal loophole for manufacturers, indicating that cross-contamination is possible.

Read labels, every single time. Products can change formulas, so even if a food is safe for you to eat one month, it may not be the next month. The best foods are the ones with labels that do not have the words "contains X."

Cooking Techniques and Tips

If you have a severe food allergy, it can be a good idea to stock your kitchen with homemade foods. Make your own stocks, sauces, seasoning mixes, and baking mixes. This is really the only way to manage a severe allergy, because you control exactly what goes into the food you eat. This may seen bothersome, but compare the time spent in the kitchen to the time you won't have to spend worrying about a reaction and getting medical help for symptoms.

Eating Out

Talk to the chef! Not the server, or the maitre d', but the chef. Quiz her extensively about the foods you want to eat, and reiterate the severity of your allergy. Make a card stating which food or foods you are allergic to, and have the chef sign it to prove he has read it. This will heighten sensitivity to your condition and may help you avoid a reaction.

Some types of restaurants are more dangerous than others. If you have a peanut or soy allergy, avoiding Chinese, Japanese, and other Asian restaurants is a good idea. Even if food you order from these restaurants doesn't contain peanuts or soy, the risk for cross-contamination is great. Avoid restaurants with buffet service. Cross-contamination risk is very high when people serve themselves. Also avoid restaurants with attached bakeries, for the same reason.

Some restaurants are intrinsically safer than others. Look for places that cook their food from scratch. Ask for recommendations from other people who have food allergies. If you've had luck with a large chain restaurant, other branches may be safe. But still be aware that chefs change their recipes. Always talk to the chef before you order from any restaurant, even one you've safely dined at before.

Hope for the Future

Currently, the only treatment for food allergies is to avoid the suspect food, in all its incarnations. Keeping an emergency kit on your person at all times is essential. But researchers are investigating possible treatments and cures that offer hope.

Researchers are working on a vaccine using genetically engineered proteins similar to those that cause the allergy but that have been changed to reduce their effect.

ALERT

Scientists hope that food allergies may be eradicated in about ten years. They are currently working on many treatments that appear promising, so there is hope for the future. In the meantime, read labels, be prepared, and try to relax and enjoy life, knowing that you can take care of yourself.

Researchers have found that mice bred to have a peanut allergy were missing a crucial molecule called Interlukin-12. This study has also shown that with peanut allergies, some of the immune cells last longer, which can provoke the immune system into a reaction. Interlukin-12 may be the missing factor that helps subdue this reaction.

Outgrowing Allergies

Many people can outgrow their food allergies, with the exception of allergies to peanuts and tree nuts. Scientists think that avoiding the problematic food for years may "reset" your body's immune system. Or, it may be that the immune system in the digestive tract matures and no longer reacts to that protein or proteins.

Children with allergies to soy, egg, milk, and wheat can outgrow their allergies; about 85 percent are no longer allergic at the age of five. Peanut allergies are usually lifelong, but 20 percent of children do outgrow it.

Preventing Allergies

No one is sure why people develop food allergies. Some studies suggest that if food allergies run in a family, pregnant women should avoid those foods while they are pregnant and nursing. Other studies have found there is no effect. The exception to this is peanuts. If there is a strong peanut allergy in your family, avoid peanuts while pregnant and nursing.

To help prevent food allergies, breastfeed your child until he is six months old, and avoid feeding him solid foods until that age. Add cow's milk to his diet after he is one year old, and introduce eggs only after the age of two. Add seafood and nuts to his diet when he is three years old, and be sure to add foods gradually as he grows. Introducing one new food at a time, waiting for a couple of weeks in between each introduction, will help you identify the food if he is allergic to it.

CHAPTER 17

Home Cooking

The convenience of restaurants, take-out, packaged and pre-prepared foods is becoming all too appealing to families across America. It makes sense, considering how little time most people have available to prepare home-cooked meals. However, today the need for home cooking is greater than ever. The average person consumes triple the amount of calories when eating out. Packaged foods are filled with preservatives, toxins, and chemicals, and we are unfamiliar with many of the ingredients. You don't have to spend hours cooking nutritious meals from scratch. In fact, the majority of the recipes in this book can be prepared in thirty minutes or less. This chapter will inspire you to devote time to preparing some good old-fashioned foods for delicious and nutritious meals.

Importance of Cooking at Home

Cooking food at home is the single most important thing you can do for your health and your family's. When you do the cooking, you have control. You know exactly what everyone is eating. You control the quality and quantity, and you can cook to meet everyone's needs and preferences. You can also be sure of the cleanliness of the facility.

Cooking at home (from scratch using fresh ingredients—not microwaving a frozen dinner) means the meal is fresher, which is a great start to obtaining more nutrients. You can maximize nutritional value by the cooking methods you use and by picking quality fresh foods without preservatives.

Eating out is fun, but it gets expensive. Home cooking using raw ingredients is not only healthier, it's also much cheaper. And you may find that cooking is just as much fun as dining out, as well as being rewarding and even therapeutic. No one says you need to make a feast fit for a king. Simple dishes and simple preparations, including the ones in this book, are easy and satisfying.

Finally, there is no better way to show you care than to cook a healthy meal for your loved ones. This nurturing act creates an enduring legacy. If you cook for your kids, they are more likely to cook for theirs, and so on. Good nutrition is a fantastic family tradition to pass on to future generations.

Healthy Cooking Methods

Preparation can dramatically affect the nutrient content of food. Cooking in a healthful way doesn't take much effort, but it does require some attention.

Broiling and grilling are known as dry-heat methods. They require no moisture, and little or no oil is necessary. Definitions vary, but grilling generally refers to food placed over a heat source, and broiling places food under a heat source.

The key to the success of dry-heat cooking is high heat. High temperatures seal the outside of the meat and hold in the juices. Lower temperatures allow more of the natural juices to drip out, yielding a drier finished product.

Stir-frying and pan frying require a small amount of oil. When using this method to cook vegetables, the high heat limits the nutrient loss and keeps the colors fresh and bright.

Steaming is a moist-heat method. Food is suspended in a basket or perforated pan over simmering water, and the heat of the steam does the cooking. Nutrients are not lost in the water as happens during boiling. They can, however, dissipate into the air if overcooked.

ESSENTIAL

Poaching is great for delicate sausages, fish filets, quenelles, and delicate fruits. The liquid used can be flavored with herbs, spices, or aromatic vegetables, but it is meant strictly for cooking, and is not generally consumed.

Food can also be steamed in its own juices by wrapping it in foil or parchment paper and baking it in the oven. This is a particularly great way to maintain moisture and flavor for low-fat meats, chicken, and fish.

Roasting is an all-around dry-heat technique that may or may not involve added fat. Roasting meat is an excellent way to eliminate fat. Because the meat is suspended on a rack above a roasting pan, the meat juices drip away.

Roasting is a great method for cooking certain vegetables, including potatoes in their jackets, onions and garlic in their skins, and squash and pumpkin still in the rind. These foods essentially steam themselves soft, and their natural sugars concentrate, providing more natural flavor than when they are peeled and boiled.

Poaching is a moist-heat method. It is not boiling, but it's close. Water is kept just below the simmer so the food is not agitated by the motion of a rolling boil. Boiling employs water or another liquid brought to a rolling boil. Simmering cooks the food under the boil, but still in motion. Food is cooked to the desired doneness.

Boiling not only increases the temperature of the cooking, but it keeps the food in motion. This is important for foods that tend to stick, such as pasta. Because boiling leaches nutrients into the cooking liquid, it is best reserved for recipes that utilize the cooking liquid, such as soups and stews.

Frugal chefs have been known to save cooking liquid for use in subsequent recipes. Stewing is another moist-heat method, and it usually involves a longer cooking time. Stews frequently feature a liquid that thickens into a sauce as part of the meal.

ESSENTIAL

Stews are often enriched with fat or starch, and in most cases they include fatty meats. That's because this method works miraculously to soften the connective tissues of tough meats and melt away the fats, turning them into succulent tender delicacies.

Shopping Strategies

Believe it or not, grocery shopping can be fun—if you are prepared and allot enough time for it, that is. It can also be a successful way to bring the entire family on board the healthy food express. Make them a part of the process and they are more likely to enjoy the changes.

Menu Planning

It may sound like a lot of work, and a little hyper-organized, but by planning out a week's worth of meals you will actually save time and money and eliminate a good deal of stress.

The first step is to brainstorm with your family for meal ideas. If they don't like it, they probably won't eat it. This is most important when it comes to snacking. If everything in the kitchen looks unappetizing, your family will find their snacks somewhere else.

After you have decided on recipes you like, make a list of all the week's meals, including breakfast, lunch, dinner, snacks, and dessert. Use it to make your list of ingredients. Whittle that list into the things you actually need to buy, then you're off to the races. (If you're a coupon clipper, don't forget your coupons!)

Bring at least one helper to the market, if you can. Kids will need lessons in label reading and price comparison. It may take a few trips until it sinks in, but persevere. Your goal is to teach them how to recognize the good from the bad. Be patient, and know that you are giving them valuable life skills.

Shopping Lists

Nutrition begins at the grocery store. More than 15,000 new food products are introduced each year, so shopping lists have changed in many ways. In addition, the media offers an abundance of conflicting information about what is healthy and what is not. It can be a challenge to understand ingredient list misconceptions and marketing gimmicks of health claims located on food packaging, so you know what to actually purchase. To help support healthy choices for the family you need to:

- Shop differently.
- Shop regularly.

A supermarket is designed to get you to buy things you don't necessarily need. Some ways supermarkets are set up against you include:

1. Milk on one side, produce on another. You have to go through the entire store to get some basic items. On your way to those locations you usually see the deli/bakery. Sometimes the smells coming from the bakery can be hard to resist.
2. The meat counter is against the entire back wall, so every time you leave an aisle you run into it. Chicken and fish are usually found at either end.
3. Often snacking items, such as candy and chips, are on one side of an aisle where a basic item, such as water, is on the other.
4. Bins of sale items are located right near the cash register to help increase impulse buying.
5. Coupon machines are placed in front of certain items.
6. High-sugar, low-fiber cereals are positioned on the lower shelves to attract kids.

What are some things you can do to tame the supermarket?

1. Check sales flyers so you know what is on sale ahead of time and are not pushed into an impulse buy because it is a good deal.
2. If you clip coupons, only do so for items you really need and use.
3. Make a list and stick to it. Double-checking your items will support healthy behaviors.
4. Don't go shopping when you're hungry.
5. Give yourself adequate time. If you rush, you'll revert to your old habits.

The best way to create a shopping list is to choose seven recipes, one for each night of the week, plus three breakfasts and lunches to alternate between days. After you've chosen your recipes, sit down and use the following form to create your shopping list. It's a good idea to save your shopping lists for future reference. Practice makes perfect!

▼ Grocery List

Fruit	Lean Proteins	Whole Grains	Fluids	Snacks

Key items to have on hand for last-minute meal prep should hold an important presence in your pantry and freezer. Proteins that fit into this category include frozen chicken breasts, shrimp, scallops, and fish fillets. You can also keep cans of beans on hand for a easy-prep grilled vegetable-bean burrito night. Eggs are great for a breakfast-for-dinner night cooked over-easy, scrambled, made into omelets, or baked into a crustless quiche. Plant proteins, such as all-natural peanut butter, nuts, soy beans, tofu, tempeh, and veggie burgers, are also great to keep in stock.

Always have frozen vegetables that can be easily pulled from the freezer to pair with one of the proteins discussed above. This way you have no excuses for missing out on your veggies. Frozen pizzas with whole-wheat crusts, served with a salad or a frozen entrée with added vegetables, prevent random drive-thrus or last minute take-outs.

Each shopping trip should include a shopping basket or carriage evaluation. At least 50 percent of your items should be fruits and vegetables. Half your produce should be fresh. You should have at least two different protein sources for breakfast and lunch choices, and five different protein sources for dinners throughout the week. Lastly, there should be four different whole-grain sources from side dishes, breads, and cereals.

Recipe Modifications

Once you choose the recipes you want to make, it may be necessary to adjust them to meet your current nutritional standards. This is not difficult, and it can be quite rewarding.

Altering recipes will rarely reduce the success of a recipe, although in some cases it may take a few tries to get it where you want it. The best strategy is to change one element at a time, adding and subtracting methods that do and don't work.

Cutting Fat

Cutting fat is an easy alteration to make to any recipe. You can start by examining the raw ingredients.

Switching to leaner meat is easy. The fat content is generally displayed prominently on the packaging. You can switch to leaner beef or opt for chicken, turkey, or fish instead. Many recipes that are written for one type of meat can easily be made with another. Try turkey, salmon, or tuna burgers for a change of pace.

Oil can be used in place of butter in almost every circumstance. Olive oil is the healthiest choice, but the flavor is fairly prominent and not necessarily desirable in all circumstances. When you want a more neutral flavor, try peanut or canola oil instead. Avoid margarine. Even those with no trans fat have an elevated melting point, which leaves an unpleasant aftertaste in your mouth. Although butter contains saturated fat, it is preferable to margarine. Another way to reduce the amount of fat in a recipe is to use a nonstick pan. Nearly every style of pot or pan ever manufactured comes in a nonstick version. Take care not to use metal utensils or scrubbies, or the nonstick surface will scrape off.

Choose reduced-fat cheeses, skim milk, light sour cream, low-fat cottage cheese, and nonfat yogurt. If cholesterol is an issue for you, replace whole eggs with egg whites or egg substitutes.

Cutting Sugar and Salt

Many sugar substitutes are available today, and many measure and cook up just like refined sugar. However, few have undergone long-term study, and some can even produce unpleasant side effects. If avoiding refined sugar is your goal, consider using honey or date sugar. (Read more about sugar in Chapter 6.)

Sodium is easy to replace with salt substitutes (see recipes in Chapter 8). Eliminating it completely will take some getting used to, but it can be done successfully given time. Avoid adding salt to recipes until they hit the table to reduce the total amount of salt consumed. Reduced sodium products are plentiful, and many of your everyday salty groceries can be replaced with low-sodium counterparts. Check the labels, and compare brands.

Increasing Nutrition

Adding food with high nutritional value is a great way to improve your recipes. Increasing the amount of vegetables also increases the vitamins, minerals, and fiber. Try grating in squash, carrots, cabbage, chopped spinach, and fresh herbs to your next soup, stew, or casserole. Be sure to add these close to the end of the cooking to maximize their vitamin and mineral content.

Add dried fruits, seeds, and nuts to baked goods and grain dishes for added protein, vitamins, minerals, and omega-3 fatty acids. Sesame, flax, and walnuts are particularly healthful. Add legumes and whole grains to casseroles, soups, pasta dishes, and salads for added soluble and insoluble fiber and protein.

Pound for Pound

Certain products can, and should, be switched outright for use on a daily basis. Use whole-wheat flour instead of white all-purpose flour. Look for stone-ground organic varieties to maximize the nutritional value. You will find that your baked goods taste and look different, but take heart. You and your family will grow accustomed to the difference in short order. You may actually come to prefer it.

Go Natural

It's amazing how many ingredients called for in a recipe aren't necessary. When in doubt, use natural ingredients, and ask yourself if you could use a more natural source instead of processed ingredients called for in some recipes. Natural flavors are usually found in lemons, limes, cilantro, thyme, parsley, basil, and vinegars.

CHAPTER 18

The Importance of Exercise

Food is fuel for your body. The right sources of fuel keep your metabolism working efficiently. However, in order to preserve your lean body mass, physical activity is needed; this sustains your overall health and increases your functional health as you age. Your mental and physical health rely on physical activity, so start moving your body. As the old saying goes, use it or lose it. The key is to choose activities you enjoy. There's an activity for everyone: playing competitive sports, biking, hiking, swimming, walking, yoga, dancing, and so on.

Your Exercise Requirement

The American Heart Association recommends thirty minutes of aerobic physical activity a day at moderate intensity. Unfortunately, this guideline is misleading.

In 1995 the Centers for Disease Control and Prevention (CDC) and the American College of Sports Medicine (ACSM) made a public health recommendation that every U.S. adult should accumulate thirty minutes or more of moderate-intensity physical activity on most, preferably all, days of the week.

The recommendation seemed clear enough, but was misinterpreted by many. Some believed that higher-intensity activity would not be beneficial; others considered it to mean that any movement would suffice. Therefore, in 2007 the following new guidelines were issued:

Healthy adults age eighteen to sixty-five need moderate-intensity aerobic physical activity of at least thirty minutes per session on five or more days per week, or vigorous-intensity aerobic activity for at least twenty minutes three or more days per week. Combinations of moderate- and vigorous-intensity activity can be performed to satisfy these requirements. In addition, every adult should perform activities that maintain or increase muscular strength and endurance a minimum of two days each week.

In order to understand these guidelines fully, it is important to understand what constitutes moderate and vigorous intensity.

Target Heart Rate

The difficulty in determining the intensity of exercise lies in the fact that everyone is different. What makes one person huff and puff will barely break a sweat on someone else. To adequately measure intensity, the target heart rate is used.

Measuring target heart rate first requires knowing your average maximum heart rate, which is determined by subtracting your age from 220. Your target heart rate is 50–85 percent of your maximum. It is a wide range. When you begin an exercise program, your target is the lower end of the range, and as you become more physically fit, you aim higher.

ALERT

Some high-blood-pressure medications can lower your maximum heart rate. Check with your doctor to determine if your medication does this, and to find your new target heart rate.

Begin by measuring your pulse. To do this, put two fingers, preferably your second and third fingers, on your carotid or radial artery. The carotid artery is alongside your windpipe, and your radial artery can be found in the groove of your inner wrist, below your thumb. Move your fingers around until you feel the pulse. Using a timepiece with a second hand or a stop watch, count the pulse beats for ten seconds. Multiply by six for your beats per minute (bpm). (Alternatively, you can count for six seconds and multiply by ten.)

▼ **Target Heart Rate**

Age	Target Heart Rate (50–85 percent)	Average Maximum Heart Rate (100 percent)
20	100–179 bpm	200 bpm
30	89–162 bpm	190 bpm
40	90–153 bpm	180 bpm
50	85–145 bpm	170 bpm
60	80–136 bpm	160 bpm
70	75–128 bpm	150 bpm

It is possible to estimate intensity without the heart rate. It's called the chat test, and it is useful if your activity doesn't allow you to take your pulse. If you can chat easily during your activity, your intensity is low. If you can speak, but are breathing heavily, your intensity is moderate. If you can't talk at all, your intensity is high.

Body Mass Index

The body mass index (BMI) is a measurement used to determine relative body fat. The number will indicate if a person is normal weight, underweight, overweight, or obese. The BMI measurement uses weight and height in its calculation and is therefore not a method that directly measures fat. Other methods, including underwater weighing and skin fold thickness measurements, are more accurate but are also more costly. BMI provides a reliable approximation and will indicate if an individual has serious body fat issues. Then, the lifestyle can be adjusted accordingly.

To measure your BMI, multiply your weight (in pounds) by 703, then divide by your height (in inches) twice:

weight (lbs.) × 703 / height (inches) / height (inches)

▼ **Body Mass Index**

BMI	Weight Status
< 18.5	underweight
18.5–24.9	normal weight
25.0–29.9	overweight
> 30.0	obese

Keep in mind that BMI is affected by several variables, including age, sex, race, and musculature. Older adults and women tend to have more body fat, whereas athletes tend to have heavy muscles. For that reason, a twenty-year-old male athlete may have the same BMI as a forty-year-old female office worker, but they may be miles apart in terms of actual fitness. The measurement is meant only as a general indication.

Weighing Your Risk

Most people already know if they are at their ideal weight. You can see it in the mirror. But you can get a more accurate indication of how your current weight stacks up to your ideal weight.

First, determine your body frame size. Medium-frame males have a seven-inch wrist. Medium-frame women have a six-inch wrist. Larger frames have larger wrists, and smaller frames have smaller wrists. Now add up the pounds to determine your ideal weight:

MEDIUM-FRAME MALES

- 100 pounds for the first five feet of height
- 5 pounds for every inch over five feet
- Take away 5 pounds for every inch under five feet

MEDIUM-FRAME FEMALES

- 106 pounds for the first five feet of height
- 6 pounds for every inch over five feet
- Take away 6 pounds for every inch under five feet
- Smaller frames subtract 10 percent
- Larger frames add 10 percent

Weigh the Results

Now that you have a general idea of where you stand, you can begin to adjust your diet accordingly. To lose weight, your calorie intake must be less than your current daily caloric needs. To gain weight, it must be more.

To lose weight (which is the more common goal), you need to burn about 3,500 calories more than you consume. So to lose one pound you must burn 3,500 calories over the course of a week, or about 500 calories per day. This can be accomplished by eliminating these calories from your diet, burning more calories through exercise, or both. For example, walking fast (so you're breathing heavily) for fifteen to twenty miles a week will burn about 2,500 calories. As your fitness improves, you must increase the intensity or duration of your exercise to maintain the weight loss.

ESSENTIAL

Keep challenging yourself. Taking the same walk day after day will only help you for so long. As your body becomes accustomed to the motion, and your muscles develop, the movement is no longer challenging, and your heart is no longer working hard. Pick up the pace, take a hill, or start running.

Water and Exercise

Unless you're an elite athlete, water is the best way to replenish fluids lost during exercise. Sports drinks are made to replenish lost electrolytes and provide added carbohydrates to fuel athletes after prolonged vigorous exercise. Everyday moderate exercise of thirty to forty minutes does not qualify.

Thirty minutes before you go out for your daily routine, drink one to two cups of water. Throughout your exercise, drink one-half to one cup of water every ten to fifteen minutes. When you're done, replenish your fluids by slowly drinking water over the next several hours. To adequately rehydrate, you should consume two cups of water for every pound lost during exercise.

Food as Fuel

Athletes are keenly aware of the fuel aspect of food, especially when it's running out. And they are familiar with the instant rejuvenation a little fuel can give when they're running on empty.

Pre-Exercise: Food That Gets You Going

Eating before an exercise routine is essential, but it should be planned carefully. Too much food too close to the activity can give you nausea, cramps, or worse. The sloshing feeling in your stomach can also be distracting. It's best to allow your food time to digest.

The best pre-exercise eating plan begins two to three hours prior to the activity. A light meal high in complex carbohydrates and some protein is ideal. A bowl of cereal, a peanut butter sandwich, a baked potato with cottage cheese, or a bagel are good choices. Avoid fat, because it is hard to digest, and it stays in the stomach longer.

Thirty to sixty minutes prior to your workout have a piece of fruit or an energy bar. These last-minute carbohydrates can help boost energy to get you started. Some athletes take a bite of simple sugar foods just before heading out the door. Experiment with this, because some people cannot handle the spike and dip in blood glucose during their sport.

So, how much food do you actually need for your workout?

- Calorie needs for training vary, but they generally hover around 17–20 calories per pound for maintenance, and 16–17 calories per pound to lose body fat.
- Protein needs for training range between 0.5 and 0.6 grams per pound. Carbohydrate needs for training are 3–5 grams per pound, and more for higher-intensity endurance sports.
- Fat needs for training are about 0.5 grams per pound, or the balance of your calories after protein and carbohydrates.
- Fluid needs for training vary too, but are generally 1 quart (32 ounces) for every 1,000 calories, plus additional fluid for exercise, from 2–5 quarts depending on the intensity.
- Caffeine before exercise is not recommended. It is a diuretic, which can cause dehydration. It can also cause nausea, muscle tremors, or headaches. The effects depend on your personal habits, and your level of addiction.

During Exercise: Electrolytes and Carbs

The electrolytes sodium and potassium are salts that can carry an electrical charge. Your cells rely on them to carry impulses for muscles and nerves. You get plenty of electrolytes in your food, so regular daily exercise does not require electrolyte replacement. But with constant, vigorous activity for more than an hour, as in long-distance running, electrolyte replacement can be beneficial.

ESSENTIAL

Endurance athletes need more than the boost they get from a sports drink. Carbohydrate gels, candy, and even soda pop are common mid-event glucose boosters. The burst of energy they provide helps delay the "bonk." Elite athletes will sometimes pop a glucose pill close to the finish line for an extra edge.

The sports drink phenomenon of today began in the 1960s with a football coach at the University of Florida. He was concerned that his athletes ran out of energy during practices. University doctors came up with a beverage that combines sodium, potassium, and carbohydrate with water to combat the loss of vital fluid in the Florida heat. The drink was a success, and soon teams from all over the country were ordering the Florida Gator's drink. Today, it is on the sidelines of every major sporting event as Gatorade.

Sports drinks are everywhere, and they are marketed relentlessly. But there is no reason to consume these high-calorie, high-sodium drinks on a regular basis. It is certainly not something to drink simply to quench thirst.

If you are a serious athlete, sip a sports drink every fifteen to thirty minutes throughout your activity to maintain a constant energy level. Look for a sports drink with a low level of fructose. This sugar causes bloating and cramping in some people and can delay water absorption, which makes exercise feel harder.

After Exercise: Food for Recuperation

Exercise takes its toll on the body. Athletes are often injured, and the body's motions wear away at joints, bones, connective tissues, and muscles. Proper nutrition is vital to immediate recovery from exercise as well as for long-term strength and stamina.

After exercise, fluid is the first thing your body wants and needs. Drink twenty to twenty-four ounces for every pound lost during your exercise session (this requires you weighing yourself before and after). Within the first fifteen minutes after exercise, ingest some carbohydrates to begin restoring glycogen. Drinking a glass of orange juice is perfect.

Muscle glycogen synthesis, the conversion of carbohydrate to glycogen for your muscles, is greater immediately after exercise, and for about forty-five minutes. Within that time frame you should consume 100–200 grams of carbohydrates. This immediately begins to rebuild your glycogen stores for later. After two hours your body's ability to convert carbohydrate to glycogen is reduced by 50 percent.

Protein is also needed after exercise to begin rebuilding muscle tissue damaged by the wear and tear of your sport. In addition, protein helps increase water absorption, which improves muscle hydration. Consume 25–50 grams of protein within the forty-five-minute window.

This 4:1 ratio of carbohydrates to protein, plus water, is easier to digest, and faster to absorb, when taken in liquid form. Smoothies and specially formulated sports drinks are ideal.

Sport Food Myths

Plenty of sports nutrition information is available, and much of it is sound. But often, what you hear in the locker room is less reliable. Here are a few commonly held beliefs that are no longer considered valid:

Myth: Eating More Protein Speeds Muscle Building and Increases Strength

Although amino acids do build muscle, and athletes should eat more protein than non-athletes, it is not possible to build muscle or strength by eating more protein. Your body will burn what it needs for energy and store the rest as fat.

Myth: Athletes Need More Vitamins for Energy

Vitamins do not provide energy; calories do. Vitamins are in the food you eat. Athletes need the same amount of vitamins as everyone else.

Myth: Athletes Need Extra Sodium and Potassium to Replace Sweat Loss

Only during extreme physical exertion do athletes lose sodium and potassium. During regular exercise it is only necessary to take in fluid, which helps keep the salts in balance.

Myth: Skipping Breakfast Helps Burn More Fat

Skipping a meal will result in fewer calories burned overall. That's because you will get tired faster and won't be working at your usual potential.

Myth: Carb Loading the Night Before an Activity Gives You More Energy

Carbohydrate loading is intended as part of a long process of building glycogen stores. It should be ongoing throughout the athlete's training, which includes the "taper," a reduction of exertion paired with an increase in carbohydrate intake during the last week before a big event.

Meal Plans

Monday

Breakfast
1 cup Greek yogurt, ½ cup dry high-fiber/low-sugar cereal, 1 sliced peach, and ¼ cup of blueberries

Snack
Sliced pear with cinnamon and stevia

Lunch
4 ounces of tuna mixed with Greek yogurt in a pita pocket with sliced tomato, cucumber, mixed greens, and avocado slice, served with 1 cup of grapes

Snack
2 tablespoons of hummus served with carrots, celery, and bell peppers

Dinner
Turkey or vegetarian chili over a baked potato with a dollop of Greek yogurt and a side of steamed broccoli

Tuesday

Breakfast
1 egg (poached, fried, or scrambled), 1 whole-wheat English muffin, and 1 slice of tomato served with an apple

Snack
¼ cup of almonds and a plum

Lunch
Turkey meatballs over spaghetti squash with steamed green beans

Snack
2 celery stalks and 2 Laughing Cow cheese wedges (add 5 sliced olives, optional)

Dinner
Veggie burger on a whole-wheat bun served with stir-fried veggies, mixed greens, and sweet potato fries

Wednesday

Breakfast
2 whole-grain waffles topped with 1 tablespoon of natural peanut butter or almond butter and banana slices

Snack
⅓ cup of cottage cheese and ½ cup of pineapple

Lunch
Whole-wheat tortilla wrap with 1 tablespoon hummus, ½ cup of tofu, lettuce, sliced tomatoes, low-fat feta cheese, and olives

Snack
¼ cup healthy nut trail mix with carrot sticks

Dinner
1 cup of marinated tofu stir-fried with vegetables and 1 cup of whole-wheat couscous

Snack
Fruit kebob

Thursday

Breakfast
¾ cup high-fiber/low-sugar cereal, 1 cup skim milk or almond milk, and 1 cup blueberries

Snack
1 cup Greek yogurt with ½ teaspoon of organic honey and 1 teaspoon of ground flaxseeds

Lunch
2 tablespoons natural peanut butter with ½ banana in a whole-grain roll-up served with 1 cup of carrots

Snack
1 serving of whole-grain crackers, 1 ounce low-fat cottage cheese, and cucumber slices

Dinner
4 ounces grilled chicken, 2 cups of vegetables, and 1 cup cooked whole-grain pasta

Friday

Breakfast
Sliced banana, ½ cup oatmeal, ¼ cup nuts

Snack
Baked apple in the microwave with cinnamon

Lunch
½ cup of low-fat cottage cheese over mixed greens with 1 cup of bell peppers, ¼ avocado, scallions, ½ cup of corn, 1 teaspoon of olive oil, ¼ cup of pumpkin seeds

Snack

1 tablespoon of SunButter with an apple

Dinner

6 ounces of broiled haddock with a baked potato, 1–2 cups of stewed tomatoes, and spinach

Saturday

Breakfast

Scrambled egg and broccoli with turkey sausage (al fresco) and sweet potato wedges

Snack

Grapefruit half with a whole-grain cracker and ¼ cup of low-fat cottage cheese

Lunch

Whole-wheat pita stuffed with vegetarian refried beans, salsa, lettuce, slice of avocado, and 1 ounce of chicken served with mixed green salad

Snack

1 tablespoon of natural peanut butter or almond butter with celery sticks and 1 tablespoon of sesame seeds

Dinner

6 ounces of scallops stir-fried with sugar snap peas, water chestnuts, and onions, served over 1 cup of cooked quinoa

Sunday

Breakfast
Whole-wheat tortilla burrito with one egg, peppers, onions, and ¼ cup low-fat cheese topped with salsa and black beans

Snack
1 cup Greek yogurt with ½ cup blueberries

Lunch
1 cup of cooked brown rice with shrimp/chicken and mixed vegetables

Snack
¼ cup of nuts and 1 cup of melon

Dinner
4 ounces grilled swordfish, 2 cups of grilled vegetables, and 1 cup cooked bulgur

Snack
Grilled fruit kebob

APPENDIX B

Body Mass Index Chart

BMI

Body weight (pounds)

Height (inches)	19	20	21	22	23	24	25	26	27	28	29	30	31	32	33	34	35	36	37	38	39	40	41	42	43	44	45	46	47	48	49	50	51	52	53	54
58	91	96	100	105	110	115	119	124	129	134	138	143	148	153	158	162	167	172	177	181	186	191	196	201	205	210	215	220	224	229	234	239	244	248	253	258
59	94	99	104	109	114	119	124	128	133	138	143	148	153	158	163	168	173	178	183	188	193	198	203	208	212	217	222	227	232	237	242	247	252	257	262	267
60	97	102	107	112	118	123	128	133	138	143	148	153	158	163	168	174	179	184	189	194	199	204	209	215	220	225	230	235	240	245	250	255	261	266	271	276
61	100	106	111	116	122	127	132	137	143	148	153	158	164	169	174	180	185	190	195	201	206	211	217	222	227	232	238	243	248	254	259	264	269	275	280	285
62	104	109	115	120	126	131	136	142	147	153	158	164	169	175	180	186	191	196	202	207	213	218	224	229	235	240	246	251	256	262	267	273	278	284	289	295
63	107	113	118	124	130	135	141	146	152	158	163	169	175	180	186	191	197	203	208	214	220	225	231	237	242	248	254	259	265	270	278	282	287	293	299	304
64	110	116	122	128	134	140	145	151	157	163	169	174	180	186	192	197	204	209	215	221	227	232	238	244	250	256	262	267	273	279	285	291	296	302	308	314
65	114	120	126	132	138	144	150	156	162	168	174	180	186	192	198	204	210	216	222	228	234	240	246	252	258	264	270	276	282	288	294	300	306	312	318	324
66	118	124	130	136	142	148	155	161	167	173	179	186	192	198	204	210	216	223	229	235	241	247	253	260	266	272	278	284	291	297	303	309	315	322	328	334
67	121	127	134	140	146	153	159	166	172	178	185	191	198	204	211	217	223	230	236	242	249	255	261	268	274	280	287	293	299	306	312	319	325	331	338	344
68	125	131	138	144	151	158	164	171	177	184	190	197	203	210	216	223	230	236	243	249	256	262	269	276	282	289	295	302	308	315	322	328	335	341	348	354
69	128	135	142	149	155	162	169	176	182	189	196	203	209	216	223	230	236	243	250	257	263	270	277	284	291	297	304	311	318	324	331	338	345	351	358	365
70	132	139	146	153	160	167	174	181	188	195	202	209	216	222	229	236	243	250	257	264	271	278	285	292	299	306	313	320	327	334	341	348	355	362	369	376
71	136	143	150	157	165	172	179	186	193	200	208	215	222	229	236	243	250	257	265	272	279	286	293	301	308	315	322	329	338	343	351	358	365	372	379	386
72	140	147	154	162	169	177	184	191	199	206	213	221	228	235	242	250	258	265	272	279	287	294	302	309	316	324	331	338	346	353	361	368	375	383	390	397
73	144	151	159	166	174	182	189	197	204	212	219	227	235	242	250	257	265	272	280	288	295	302	310	318	325	333	340	348	355	363	371	378	386	393	401	408
74	148	155	163	171	179	186	194	202	210	218	225	233	241	249	256	264	272	280	287	295	303	311	319	326	334	342	350	358	365	373	381	389	396	404	412	420
75	152	160	168	176	184	192	200	208	216	224	232	240	248	256	264	272	279	287	295	303	311	319	327	335	343	351	359	367	375	383	391	399	407	415	423	431
76	156	164	172	180	189	197	205	213	221	230	238	246	254	263	271	279	287	295	304	312	320	328	336	344	353	361	369	377	385	394	402	410	418	426	435	443

Normal   Overweight   Obese   Extreme Obesity

Standard U.S./Metric Measurement Conversions

VOLUME CONVERSIONS

U.S. Volume Measure	Metric Equivalent
⅛ teaspoon	0.5 milliliters
¼ teaspoon	1 milliliters
½ teaspoon	2 milliliters
1 teaspoon	5 milliliters
½ tablespoon	7 milliliters
1 tablespoon (3 teaspoons)	15 milliliters
2 tablespoons (1 fluid ounce)	30 milliliters
¼ cup (4 tablespoons)	60 milliliters
⅓ cup	90 milliliters
½ cup (4 fluid ounces)	125 milliliters
⅔ cup	160 milliliters
¾ cup (6 fluid ounces)	180 milliliters
1 cup (16 tablespoons)	250 milliliters
1 pint (2 cups)	500 milliliters
1 quart (4 cups)	1 liter (about)

WEIGHT CONVERSIONS

U.S. Weight Measure	Metric Equivalent
½ ounce	15 grams
1 ounce	30 grams
2 ounces	60 grams
3 ounces	85 grams
¼ pound (4 ounces)	115 grams
½ pound (8 ounces)	225 grams
¾ pound (12 ounces)	340 grams
1 pound (16 ounces)	454 grams

OVEN TEMPERATURE CONVERSIONS

Degrees Fahrenheit	Degrees Celsius
200 degrees F	100 degrees C
250 degrees F	120 degrees C
275 degrees F	140 degrees C
300 degrees F	150 degrees C
325 degrees F	160 degrees C
350 degrees F	180 degrees C
375 degrees F	190 degrees C
400 degrees F	200 degrees C
425 degrees F	220 degrees C
450 degrees F	230 degrees C

BAKING PAN SIZES

American	Metric
8 x 1½ inch round baking pan	20 x 4 cm cake tin
9 x 1½ inch round baking pan	23 x 3.5 cm cake tin
1 x 7 x 1½ inch baking pan	28 x 18 x 4 cm baking tin
13 x 9 x 2 inch baking pan	30 x 20 x 5 cm baking tin
2 quart rectangular baking dish	30 x 20 x 3 cm baking tin
15 x 10 x 2 inch baking pan	30 x 25 x 2 cm baking tin (Swiss roll tin)
9 inch pie plate	22 x 4 or 23 x 4 cm pie plate
7 or 8 inch springform pan	18 or 20 cm springform or loose bottom cake tin
9 x 5 x 3 inch loaf pan	23 x 13 x 7 cm or 2 lb narrow loaf or pate tin
1½ quart casserole	1.5 litre casserole
2 quart casserole	2 litre casserole

Index

We Have

EVERYTHING®

on Anything!

With more than 19 million copies sold, **the Everything® series** has become one of America's favorite resources for solving problems, learning new skills, and organizing lives. Our brand is not only recognizable—it's also welcomed.

The series is a hand-in-hand partner for people who are ready to tackle new subjects—like you!

For more information on the Everything® series, please visit *www.adamsmedia.com*

The Everything® list spans a wide range of subjects, with more than 500 titles covering 25 different categories:

Business	History	Reference
Careers	Home Improvement	Religion
Children's Storybooks	Everything Kids	Self-Help
Computers	Languages	Sports & Fitness
Cooking	Music	Travel
Crafts and Hobbies	New Age	Wedding
Education/Schools	Parenting	Writing
Games and Puzzles	Personal Finance	
Health	Pets	